Health systems and public health medicine in the European Community

Mark McCarthy

Sian Rees

AF849197

FACULTY OF PUBLIC HEALTH MEDICINE
of the Royal Colleges of Physicians of the UK
and
ROYAL COLLEGE OF PHYSICIANS OF LONDON

The Authors

Mark McCarthy, MA, MSc, MB BChir, PhD, MRCP, FFPHM, studied at the University of Cambridge, University College, London, and the London School of Economics. He is currently Director of Public Health, Camden and Islington, and Honorary Senior Lecturer, University College, London.

Sian Rees, BA, MB BS, MSc, studied at the University of Oxford and University College, London. She is currently Senior Registrar in Public Health Medicine, North-West Thames Region and Charing Cross and Westminster Medical School.

Royal College of Physicians of London
11 St Andrews Place, London NW1 4LE

Copyright © 1992 Mark McCarthy and Sian Rees
ISBN 1 873240 44 9

Typeset by Oxprint Ltd
Printed by The Lavenham Press Ltd,
Lavenham, Sudbury, Suffolk

Foreword

Public Health Medicine has always been concerned with major issues and problems that affect the health of society as a whole. Within Europe, developments in public health and, in particular, the role of medical practitioners have been very varied. In its narrowest sense, public medicine can be taken simply as an endeavour to avert the development of disease; in its broadest as a positive programme of health maintenance.

The beginnings of concern with public health appeared with the publication of the first vital and health statistics by John Graunt in 1662, and the acceptance across Europe by the mid-eighteenth century that morbidity and mortality were not of supernatural origin. Jules Guerin introduced the term 'social medicine' in France in 1848 when he appealed to the French medical profession to act in the public interest and help to create the new society for which the French Revolution had prepared the ground. Since John Simon's intensive research into the causes of disease and death, in the late nineteenth century, epidemiology has been instrumental in basing the practice of public health on fact rather than supposition.

Yet, although the role of public health medicine has been accepted in all countries in Europe, its definition, scope and the skills required have not been widely discussed on an international level. The World Health Organisation has played a major role in promoting public health medicine world-wide, but in some countries the concepts remain restricted to environmental factors that were of importance in the 19th and at the beginning of the 20th century. In other countries the tasks of medical practitioners in public health have been subsumed by managers or non-medical workers concerned primarily with the efficient administration of services or institutions, or perhaps with simplistic concepts of altering behaviour or the environment.

The importance of public health, and the opportunities for its improvement created within the European Community, were discussed at a meeting of individuals from each of the member countries, convened by the Faculty of Public Health Medicine with the help of The Nuffield Provincial Hospitals Trust. This book gives an account of the health systems for each member state and thus provides the framework within which public health medicine will develop. It is thus a landmark in the development of European Public Medicine and also provides a guide to the training and educational requirements for our countries.

WALTER W. HOLLAND
President
Faculty of Public Health Medicine

Contents

Preface

Integration within the European Community (EC) is developing with increasing speed. The Treaty on European Union, agreed at the Maastricht summit of December 1991, has brought closer political and military co-operation to the head of the EC's agenda. The Single Market Act is set to be in place by the end of 1992. While the United Kingdom rejected the social chapter from the draft Treaty, and it is clear that member states wish to retain sovereignty in the organisation of their health systems, the Maastricht summit has given legal competence for the EC to work within the field of 'public health', and the Community will now seek to formalise the management of its responsibilities and explore its new role.

At such a time, this book seeks to provide a point of reference for future debate on health care in the EC. In the first section, we describe some structural aspects of the EC and give a brief historical view of the development of health systems in Europe. In the second section we describe the health systems of each of the 12 countries of the EC as they currently stand. While each country's description may be referred to individually by the reader, we have used the same structure for each country so as to provide a basis for comparisons. A more general discussion forms the final section of the book, and draws attention to the need to develop public health medicine within the EC, making some suggestions of the path forward for this.

MARK McCARTHY
SIAN REES

Acknowledgements

We thank the Nuffield Provincial Hospitals Trust, whose board generously funded this study and the seminar on which the discussion on public health medicine is based. We must also thank the participants of the seminar held at the Nuffield Provincial Hospitals Trust in September 1991 who amended our country reports and advised us on public health medicine within their own countries. Professor Walter Holland, President of the Faculty of Public Health Medicine, initiated the project and has patiently guided us in the work. Lastly, we are grateful to Nanou Kunz and Linda Frankland for their administrative support.

MARK McCARTHY
SIAN REES

1 | Introduction

The European Community consists of 12 sovereign European states which have agreed to co-operate in defined areas of economic, social and political activity (British Medical Association 1991). Originally, there were three European Communities: the European Coal and Steel Community, established by the Treaty of Paris in 1951; the European Economic Community, established by the Treaty of Rome in 1957; and the European Atomic Energy Committee, established by the same treaty. The Merger Treaty of 1965 established a single Council and single Commission for the three communities. Since they work together, the three communities are now commonly referred to as the European Community (EC).

There are currently 12 member countries—Belgium, Denmark, France, Germany, Greece, Ireland, Italy, Luxembourg, Netherlands, Portugal, Spain and the United Kingdom (UK.). Portugal and Spain are the newest countries, and are still within the 7-year period in which countries may make any changes necessary to their legislature in order to comply with the Community Law.

Institutions

The Commission

The Commission is the executive body of the Community, developing policies and monitoring the implementation of Community legislation. The Commission seeks the opinion of the European Parliament on its proposals, but the 17 members of the Commission are nominated by member states, not by the European Parliament. The power of the Commission is its sanction to be able to take governments or businesses to the European Court of Justice at the Hague.

Council of Ministers

The Community's principal decisions are made by the Council of Ministers, which includes a representative of each national government. Legislation is proposed and drafted by the Commission. The Presidency of the Council of Ministers rotates every six months between member countries. In parallel, the 12 heads of government meet twice a year at summit meetings, termed the European Council.

Directorates-General

The Commission has 23 Directorates-General (DGs) each of which administers a general policy area. Since the original European Community Treaties did not formally include the field of health care, no individual DG was given overall responsibility for health. Health policy issues are currently addressed by several directorates, but each only partially.

- *DG III* is concerned with the internal market and industry. A section of the directorate is responsible for mutual recognition of diplomas and free movement of doctors.
- *DG V* is concerned with employment, industrial relations and social affairs. This directorate has included programmes of a general public health nature (on AIDS and cancer). It is likely that the Commission's new competence in public health, agreed in the Maastricht Treaty, will be led from this directorate.
- *DG XI* is concerned with the environment, consumer protection and nuclear safety.
- *DG XII* oversees science, research and development, including biomedical and health services research.
- *DG XIII* is responsible for telecommunication, information industries and innovation. The Advanced Informatics in Medicine (AIM) research programme is sited here.

The Single Market

In 1986 Member States signed an accord, the Single European Act, to establish a 'single market' by the end of 1992. Since health care was not formally included within the Treaty of Rome, the implications to the health sector of this agreement were not substantial: the aspects most affected were the pharmaceutical industry, laboratories, medical equipment and private health insurance.

The free movement of doctors and other health staff within the Community was agreed in directives from the Commission in 1975. Since then, a doctor may seek full registration in any member state if the doctor is a citizen of a member state, has completed primary training in a member state and holds a recognised qualification. Doctors are expected to 'acquire, in their interest and that of their patients, the linguistic knowledge necessary to the exercise of their profession in the host country', and to abide by the professional and ethical codes of the country in which they practise. Similar directives apply to other health professions—dentists, nurses, midwives and pharmacists.

Other health affairs are coming increasingly onto the Commission's agenda. First, in the field of public health, the Heads of State group have adopted two 'action plans' for AIDS and cancer. These action plans are 'decisions' binding on all member states. They are resourced and being carried out through DG V under the framework for 'social affairs'.

Second, the President of the Commission, Jacques Delors, has sought to move beyond the single economic market and create a wider 'European social dimension'. He has spoken of changing the EC from 'a community of businessmen to a community of citizens'. The Commission's proposals for a Social Charter were debated and agreed at Strasbourg in December 1989 by the heads of all member states except the UK.

Third, research within DG XII (biomedical and health services research) and DG XIII (AIM programme) is being funded to develop co-operation between member countries. In DG XII, for example, the biomedical research programme is organised through 'concerted actions'; generally they do not pay for basic staff in each country but do so for conferences and visits which bring research workers together. The research programmes must give 'added value': that is, create knowledge that could not be obtained by a single country alone.

European medical bodies

The EC set up a statutory body, the Advisory Committee for Medical Training, in 1975 with the remit

> 'to help to ensure a comparably demanding standard of medical training in the Community, with regard both to basic training and further training'.

The Committee seeks to: provide information on training methods and courses in member states; encourage discussion towards common training and performance standards; and review the adaptation of medical training to developments in medical science and teaching methods.

Each country has three representatives, one each for the national professional body, the universities and the 'competent authority' for registration (in the UK this is the General Medical Council (GMC)).

A Committee of Senior Officials in Public Health was also set up in 1975 to review implementation of the directives for mutual recognition of medical diplomas and provide information 'on the conditions under which general and specialist medical care is given in the member states'.

The main national medical professional bodies within each EC country are represented on the Permanent Committee (CP) of Doctors of the EC, established in 1959. Affiliated to this Committee, and normally working through it, are several organisations representing sectors of medical practice. The two main bodies are the European Union of Medical Specialists (UEMS), and the European Union of General Practitioners (UEMO).

The UEMS seeks to co-ordinate the work and recognition of 'monospecialties', of which 28 are currently identified. The monospecialist sections report to the Management Council. The UEMS is concerned to harmonise specialist training in member states, and has recently proposed to establish 'European Boards' for monospecialties. They are seen as providing advice for the Commission on mono-specialty training, and are not, at present, proposing to introduce European specialty examinations.

General practitioners (GPs) in Europe are represented on the UEMO. It successfully brought about a Commission directive requiring a minimum of two years training in general practice, likely to be increased to three years in 1995. Other European organisations liaising with the Standing Committee include groups representing junior hospital doctors, 'senior' hospital doctors, salaried doctors, and the Conférence International des Ordres which is concerned with registration, professional and ethical issues.

2 A brief history of health care in the European Community

Health systems, like other social institutions, are constantly evolving. Because they are the concern of everyone in a country, health systems are naturally subject to political influences which may be expressed either as demands for change or resistance to change. In all the EC countries the public profile of health care has been increasing as governments have sought to intervene in the system—usually to control rising costs.

In most countries the public hold in high regard the services provided by personal (ambulatory care) doctors and in hospitals. In Britain, social surveys over the past ten years have regularly identified health care at the top of services that the public support, and indeed show that the public would be prepared to pay more for better services. Where there is social insurance or tax-based finance for the health system, there is little public pressure to limit expenditure. Equally, doctors and others working in health care seek to expand or improve services, and are supported by pressure from an active pharmaceutical and medical technology industry. It has been the governments of all EC countries that have, to a greater or lesser extent, needed to control the health system to limit rising costs and ensure equity of provision.

The health systems of individual EC countries are the product of local political choices and national laws. Nevertheless, it is possible to suggest that a general 'European' health system exists which can be distinguished from the systems of other developed countries, for example, USA or Japan, and those of developing countries (Abel Smith 1972).

Historical research in Germany (Alber, Esping-Andersen and Rainwater 1987) has established the common thread of history in European countries. Before the nineteenth century, much health care was provided to the sick poor through charitable (often ecclesiastic) agencies. Thus, the word 'hospital' derives from hospice, a place of refuge for travellers or a place of care for the poor. During the nineteenth century traditional economic relationships changed as industrialisation developed. The towns increased in population. Associations of working men were established and received grudging legal recognition by governments, many still sovereign states with the memory of the French revolution fresh in their minds.

An important objective of many of these working men's associations was to provide mutual support for members in the event of sickness. Large families with a single wage earner (as child labour in factories became proscribed) depended heavily on the father, and sickness or injury could send the family into destitution. The mutual funds, or provident associations, were established initially to ensure income support; but they also developed methods of insuring for medical expenses, the commonest of which was for the association to retain a doctor for its members. The doctor's fees were shared among members who paid a single level of contribution whatever use they made of the service (the concept of 'solidarity'). This method also ensured that the doctor could rely on an income when providing medical services to poor people.

Yet there was a conflict of views within the medical profession on the best strategy for receiving payment. Doctors saw their economic interests differently according to the wealth of their patients. Doctors treating the poor were often poorly paid themselves, and benefited from holding a 'list' of patients for a mutual association. Doctors treating the rich could charge higher fees, see fewer patients and did not rely on mutual insurance to pay the fees. The equation of pre-paid insurance with low medical incomes and fee-for-service with higher incomes has remained a perception of doctors' leaders in the twentieth century.

As membership of the legalised mutual associations increased so did their power. State leaders, mindful also of the growth of political groupings of working people, sought ways of controlling the associations. Germany led the way, in 1883, by introducing compulsory social insurance, and several other European countries followed in the years up to the first world war. Compulsion was, however, only for 'working men', that is, those employed by others in factories or other business. People living on the land (whether landowners or peasants), living on wealth, or independent professional practitioners, were not included within the legislation.

In the twentieth century there has been a widening of social insurance legislation in all EC countries to include ever larger segments of the population and for wider areas of social provision. The most important stimulus was the extension of the voting franchise that occurred after the first world war: men who had served their country at the front could no longer be denied basic political rights. During the 1920s many European countries developed national insurance agencies with their substantial financial power held closely by the state, while the self-help associations declined. In some countries compulsory insurance was developed within economic sectors, crafts or professions, deliberately dividing working class organisations from each other and increasing control by the state. This 'corporatism' started in fascist Italy, and Germany later imposed it on several countries it occupied.

The end of the second world war in Europe offered the opportunity of a new start for social welfare. The 'total war', of families rather than men alone, had led to greater social solidarity than ever before. In Britain, the Beveridge report, seeking to overcome the 'five wants'—income, health, housing, education and social support—led a debate on post-war welfare policy. Other European countries under fascism did not have this opportunity. Moreover, in post-war elections, a socialist parliamentary majority in Britain was able to implement reforms for a 'welfare state', whereas most other countries now forming the EC voted coalitions or centre-right majorities that had no commitment to comprehensive welfare provision.

In the post-war period all EC countries have moved towards a 'welfare state', in that financing of social provision, including health care, is increasingly controlled by national laws and state ministries. There are several reasons for this. The first is the growing numbers and proportion of the population in need of services, especially older people. (This growth in numbers of older people is mainly the result of the higher birth rates at the beginning of the century rather than increased longevity.) The second reason is the rising costs of care due to new needs identified, and new skills and technology. The third reason is that 'third party' insurance lacks the mechanism of price control inherent in normal market relationships: when service providers seek to improve their incomes, insurers pass on higher costs as higher premiums without demur. (There is no evidence that private or non-profit insurance is any more able to control price inflation than insurance controlled directly by governments.)

Although the EC countries all now seek to allow access to health care according to need rather than wealth, different mechanisms have been used to achieve this, with rather different results. One country facing this problem currently is the Netherlands where about 50% of the population are insured through state insurance and 50% through private for-profit insurance companies. The state has sought to regulate people into the two alternatives according to ability to pay, but the effect has been cost-shifting from the private sector into the public sector: sick people tend to transfer into the public sector if their private insurance premiums rise. One proposal, the Dekker Report, suggested that private insurers take on the same burden of risks and level of benefits as the public sector (Ministry of Welfare 1988). The report, however, was not accepted, and a new proposal is to transfer most health insurance into the public sector.

Broadly, in most other EC countries, public regulation of health insurance and a variable contribution from taxes has led to relatively stable financing systems ensuring near universal access to comprehensive services. Over the next decade a key issue will be the extent that member states maintain risk-sharing (between people with different health status and across age groups) for their citizens or allow differential access according to wealth. Since health care 'consumption' appears to rise, rather than fall, with increasing national or personal income, the pressures for differential access may increase.

Development of the other side of health care, provision of services, will also depend strongly on government decisions. Again, risk-sharing and equity suggest the need for local access to primary care, either through GPs or clinic-based specialists, and general hospitals serving city neighbourhoods, smaller towns or rural provinces. Private medicine ('liberal' in Latin countries) will certainly continue, with regulation through professional bodies. But the opportunities for commercial providers—privately owned clinics or hospitals—is less clear. With public regulation of financing, the quest to control costs could limit the attractiveness of commercial development.

3 Health systems of the European Community countries

The health systems of European Community countries have been described in a number of previous publications. Maynard (1975) provided descriptions of the structure and financing of (then) nine EC countries, and Abel-Smith and Maynard (1979) gave more detailed descriptions of financing. Maxwell (1981) included five EC countries in his analysis of health care expenditures and McLachlan and Maynard (1982) four countries in their assessment of the private/public mix of health care provision. More recently, Field (1989) has edited a review of selected health systems around the world, Duplessis, Dab, McCarthy and Portella (1989) have edited a book describing public health services which included nine EC countries, Ham, Robinson and Benzeval (1990) have compared health organisation and financing in selected European and north American countries, and Casparie, Hermans and Paelink (1990) report a conference on financing and provision in all 12 EC countries. A recent detailed description of the Italian health service is provided by McCarthy (1992), and EC country reports and an overview of health services have been edited by Schneider, Dennerlain, Köse and Scholtes (1992).

The following descriptions have been drawn from these, and allied, publications sources, and have been supplemented by discussion with advisers from each country.

BELGIUM

Introduction

Belgium is a densely populated country of almost 10 million people covering an area of 30,518 sq km. The north and south of the country have separate languages and heritages. In the north, Flanders, Flemish is spoken (a language similar to Dutch) whilst in the south, Walloonia, French is spoken. German is spoken in some eastern parts of the country. The country has a constitutional monarchy, and an economy based on external trade.

The political structure of the country has changed considerably over the past 20 years. Power has passed from the central government to the communes, representing the linguistic and cultural groups, and the regions (Flanders, Brussels and Walloonia). The communes are responsible for social issues such as health, education and the arts, while the regions manage employment, transport and the environment. To match this devolution, the political parties have fragmented between the different cultural groups.

Health care system

Most aspects of health care are decentralised. Health policies and plans are proposed and implemented locally, while central government regulates. The Ministry of Health approves hospital building and contributes up to 75% of the construction costs. The Ministry also oversees standards of clinical practice, training and research. Belgium has one of the highest ratios of doctors to patients of all EC countries, both because there are no controls on the numbers entering training and because of the fee-for-service system of payment.

Finance

Health insurance is compulsory for almost the whole population. There are six main health insurance organisations which are federations of regional alliances of local mutual health insurance societies. Five of these federations are aligned along traditional religious and ideological lines, for example the Christian and socialist funds. The sixth, the Auxiliary Fund, is managed by the government. There are also smaller funds for certain groups such as war veterans and miners.

The National Institute for Sickness Insurance (INAMI) is the national body responsible for regulating the insurance federations. It is controlled by a board of directors which represents the mutual societies, employers and employees, hospitals and professionals. It is responsible for fee negotiations and advice to, and training for, the mutual societies. The National Office of Social Security (ONSS) collects all insurance contributions. This money, supplemented with government funds, is paid to INAMI, and thence to the federations and other health insurance associations, with a weighting according to benefits that have been paid out. At the end of the year the state makes up any losses incurred by INAMI.

People are free to enrol in whichever local mutual aid society they please. The only stipulation is that dependents must belong to the same society. An individual is free to change membership at the end of any three-month period. The contributions are split approximately one-third from the employer and two-thirds from the employee. Government subsidies for unemployed, elderly and poor people, and people with certain diseases such as tuberculosis, amount to about 30% of the funds. Compulsory insurance for the self-employed usually covers only inpatient and expensive specialist care, and supplementary ambulatory care insurance is usually purchased.

Copayments are required for about 25% of physician costs, although for some expensive outpatient or inpatient services 100% of the costs are paid directly to the provider by the insurance funds. A small daily payment is also made by patients for inpatient care. Dental services and drugs also have copayments. Other services such as home nursing, physiotherapy, glasses, hearing aids and speech therapy are usually covered by insurance if prescribed by a doctor.

Providers of health care

Hospitals

Sixty per cent of hospital beds (80% of psychiatric beds) are private not-for-profit. Private for-profit hospitals are illegal. Most private hospitals are sponsored by the Catholic church, and a few by mutual insurance societies. State hospitals include university and municipal hospitals, the latter having a board of directors (Public Assistance Commission) appointed by the city council.

Medical specialists in hospital are paid by item of service and are mainly private contractors rather than paid employees. Patients are paid the fee, minus copayment, by the insurance company. The doctor shares the fee with the hospital in proportion to their use of facilities. Higher charges are made to patients in semi-private or private rooms.

Excluding medical fees, hospitals are paid daily costs as a prospective budget. Around 25% of the total comes from central government and 75% from the insurance companies, with payment directly to the hospital. The Ministry of Health adjudicates the level of payments to different hospitals.

Ambulatory care

Patients may chose to see either a GP or specialist on first consultation, but hospital admission usually requires a specialist opinion. Most ambulatory care doctors are single-handed and in private practice, although there is a recent trend towards groups. GPs tend to work without any ancillary staff and do not have hospital attachments.

Specialists are generally grouped together in polyclinics or hospital outpatients. The polyclinics were developed by the insurance funds in the inter-war period and there are now about 265, mainly in towns. Specialists working in polyclinics are obliged to use the standard schedule of charges. Ambulatory specialists usually also have hospital staff appointments. Although there is an official schedule of prices negotiated with the insurance funds, this is a price floor—doctors are not allowed to charge below it. About one in six doctors is believed to reject this schedule completely.

Home nursing, and child health and antenatal clinics are largely organised by voluntary bodies. Up to 90% of their costs are offset by government grants.

Public health

Public health in Belgium started in the mid-nineteenth century with the establishment of Inspectors of Hygiene. However, there has been little evolution of their posts since then.

Public health medicine

There is little formal organisation of public health, mainly because of the intensely private orientation of other medical services, and subsequent lack of co-ordination. Most responsibilities of the Ministry of Health are delegated to the three regional councils. Each province has one or more health officers, usually part-time and responsible for communicable disease control, registration of births and deaths and other administrative duties. These are the only official public health doctors in the country: there are currently about 20.

Undergraduate teaching

Courses in hygiene, and sometimes epidemiology, are given in medical schools, but research in the university departments is not usually focused on health service problems.

Postgraduate training

A proportion of doctors developing an orientation towards public health have gained their experience in the colonial medical service. There is a one-year postgraduate diploma in public health, followed by a state examination. Not all the doctors holding health officer posts have had even this training, and new postgraduates find it difficult to gain appropriate employment subsequently. Further training, especially for academic posts, is often taken abroad.

DENMARK

Introduction

The population of Denmark is around 5 million. The country covers an area of 43,069 sq km and is fairly densely populated with the majority of the population living in towns or suburban areas. The country is governed as a constitutional monarchy with an elected parliament.

Within the country, Greenland and the Faroe Islands have extensive internal autonomy. There are 14 counties with an average population of 300,000, and 273 municipalities with an average population of 18,000, excluding the city of Copenhagen and the borough of Frederiksberg which have both county and municipality status.

Health care system

Health care is comprehensive in coverage and services, and publicly financed as a result of reforms in 1973 that replaced the mutual sickness funds. It is highly decentralised, with counties responsible for running and planning most health care and the municipalities being responsible for certain public health services.

The Ministry of Health has a number of other agencies beneath it, covering areas such as health promotion, research and food policy. Other ministries have some health responsibilities, for example, occupational health within the Ministry of Labour.

Planning takes place by discussion between all three levels of administration (state, counties and municipalities), although there is no formal approval procedure.

Finance

Eighty-five per cent of health expenditure is financed through county and central government taxation. The remaining 15% comes from patients' payments. The entire population is covered equally, with no insurance fees or income differentials.

Two groups of coverage are available. *Group 1* comprises 97% of the population. They receive free GP care and are free to change their GP once a year, choosing a practitioner from a given area. Consultation with a specialist requires GP referral. *Group 2* are those people that opt to pay some part of their consultation fee in order to have free access to any GP and direct specialist access. Hospital care is free for both groups. The decision as to which group to belong can be made every year.

Payment for drugs is partially covered by the national health system. There are four groups of reimbursement for drugs: no reimbursement (unless applied for by the physician on behalf of the patient), 50%, 75% and, for insulin, 100% reimbursement. Patients are repaid by the health care reimbursement scheme run by the counties. Some groups, including older people, receive free drugs.

Up to 50% of dental care payment will be reimbursed. Young people and children are entitled to free municipal dental care. There is little private health insurance, except for copayments (dentistry, drugs, glasses) and for overseas travel.

Providers of health care

Hospitals

Hospitals are run by the counties, except the University Hospital of Copenhagen which comes under the Ministry of Health. There are also five other specialist hospitals that receive national referrals, and payment is made to the county that runs the hospital by the referring county. Hospital running costs account for the largest single portion of the counties' health budgets. The finance comes from local taxes and block grants from central government. The central government support grant is weighted according to socio-economic factors such as the numbers of elderly or extent of poor housing.

The majority of hospitals are part of the public hospital service. However, in the late 1980s, a fully private, for-profit hospital was set up. More private hospitals are planned.

Hospital doctors employed by the county are full time. They provide both inpatient and outpatient care. Salaries are negotiated with representative organisations. Some specialists work in primary care, for example in ENT and ophthalmology: they often have hospital appointments as well. Otherwise, except for emergencies, patients must be referred by their GP for hospital care.

Ambulatory care

Primary health care is provided by GPs and community nurses. Any qualified physician can set up practice and has a right to private practice. However, most GPs are paid by the county through a mixture of capitation and fee-for service, and there is control of the number of physicians practising in the public service in each county.

Community nurses are divided into public health nurses—pre-school and school child health—and home nurses, who visit the elderly and infirm and provide post-treatment follow up. Since the 1970s there have been significant attempts to strengthen primary care. Health centres now exist to which nurses, laboratory workers and physiotherapists can be attached. More than 50% of GPs operate from group practices.

Municipalities are responsible for most community services, including community nursing, child health, child dental care and school health. In addition, most local services for the elderly and the running of nursing homes come under municipal jurisdiction. The cost of social services is supported by the state grants.

Public health

There is a long tradition of state employed local medical officers who deal with public health affairs. The reorganisation in 1974 led to the establishment of a medical officer of health's department in each county. These officers have a responsibility to advise on environmental health, social medicine and the health of the local population. They are also responsible for complaints processing and the certification of deaths that occur under unusual circumstances.

Public health medicine

The speciality of public health medicine was formally recognised in 1984. It consists of three branches: occupational, social and administrative medicine. The last consists primarily of those doctors who are medical officers of health. There are approximately 60 such posts across the country. Doctors working in social medicine (about 25 posts) are primarily concerned with research, teaching and policy, and are sited at the three major institutes for social medicine. Each county will have 3–4 occupational health doctors attached to hospital occupational health departments. There are also some occupational health doctors working at a national level and in academic positions.

Undergraduate teaching

The provision of basic public health education to all doctors as undergraduates has increased substantially since the mid-1980s. There are now 200 hours of teaching across six years of medical school. Subjects taught include epidemiology, environmental and occupational health, and social medicine.

Postgraduate training

This has undergone major restructuring over the past few years. All public health medicine sub-specialities require at least 18 months further clinical training after the 18 months' internship. Public health training then lasts a further three years. There is a 17-week diploma course followed by one year's research. This is common to all three sub-specialties. The diploma course has no examinations and entry is determined according to previous work experience. Although at present there is no MSc course in Denmark, the Nordic School of Public Health in Gothenburg takes Danish postgraduate students.

Training in administrative public health is then one year at a central administrative organisation and one year as a local junior medical officer of health. Occupational health is similar, with one year at a state department and one year at an occupational health clinic. Training in social medicine is concluded by two years in a municipal department of social medicine. There is little national co-ordination of training, and no formal training schemes. The National Board of Health, in conjunction with the various medical societies, approves posts.

There are public health departments at the three main medical schools. These are usually divided into social, occupational and environmental medicine. However, a large amount of public health research is carried out at the Danish Institute for Clinical Epidemiology, which is within the Ministry of Health and is funded partly by the State and partly through contracts. Although epidemiologists are usually medical doctors, academic/service links are not well developed.

FRANCE

Introduction

France is a republic of 55 million people, with a surface area of 551,000 sq km. The country borders several other EC member states. The economy is the fourth largest within the Organisation for Economic Co-operation and Development (OECD), and the country has both a wide range of natural resources as well as substantial industrial development.

There has been considerable political stability since the 1960s under a presidential system of government. Administration is traditionally centralised, with direct control by ministries of public services through prefects in 96 mainland departments. A decentralisation law, introduced in 1982, provided regional and department elected councils. However, as yet there has been only a partial shift of responsibilities from central to local administration, leading sometimes to the services being divided.

Health care system

France has an avowedly 'plural' health system, with public and private financing and provision. The Ministry of Health controls some services through regional and department prefects, while other services have parallel control through regional and department councils. The national health care funds are also divided from national to regional and local level; negotiation from providers for payment is made at all three levels, depending on the size of the provider.

Patients may refer themselves either to GPs or directly to specialists. Doctors hold strongly to the model of 'liberal practice', that is, the freedom to set their own fees, charging fees directly from patients at the time of service, and the freedom to choose their patients. This claim for independence from public control has dominated the development of the health system, although many doctors, in practice, are salaried and employed in public agencies.

Finance

Compulsory public health insurance covers almost the whole population. A single insurance fund for salaried workers includes about 78% of the population. Other funds include those for agricultural workers (9%), self-employed people (6%), and a further 15 funds together covering about 5% of the population. While they are autonomous in organisation, the funds are amalgamated at national level before distribution as 'social security'.

Both employers and employees pay social security, with contributions proportional to income. Levels of contribution are negotiated between representatives of employers, trades unions and the state, but the level is not formally agreed by parliament. The funds do not belong to the state, although the Minister of Health contributes to decisions on their use.

The funds pay for about three-quarters of health expenditures. Another one-fifth comes from copayments, paid either directly by patients or (increasingly) from secondary insurance. There are also direct payments for 'mutuelles', and from the state. The mutuelles, non-profit friendly societies which have developed in relation to specific occupational groups, are playing an increasing role. They extend levels of benefit, sometimes through directly providing services, and pay the differences between agreed levels of social security reimbursement and provider charges. Because of active marketing by the mutuelles, there is relatively little call on private for-profit health insurance.

For ambulatory care, patients usually pay their costs and are refunded by social security on a fixed rate—around 75% for medical services. The copayment ('ticket') may be refunded by the mutuelle or private insurance. There are exemptions on copayments for some chronic diseases. Drugs must also be paid for at the time of purchase, with proportional refunds: some drugs deemed of low benefit have higher copayment charges. Most inpatient, and some outpatient, charges are paid to providers directly by social security, although patients may be charged a standard fee (not usually more than 20% of the total) at the time of service.

Providers of care

Hospitals

About two-thirds of hospital beds are public, ranging from local general hospitals to regional centres. Public hospitals are required to provide a full range of services, including emergencies, and therefore are generally larger than private hospitals. Doctors can choose either setting for care of their patients, with remuneration from social security.

Public hospitals are managed by bodies established in law; these bodies may be very large (for example, the Assistance Publique de Paris), or more local. Private hospitals are owned by individuals (eg doctors) or by larger commercial companies, some operating elsewhere in the health care sector.

Remuneration is different between the two sectors. Public hospitals, and non-profit hospitals such as those run by the mutuelles, have since 1982 received an annual cash-limited prospective budget. Private hospitals remain reimbursed on cost-per-day with a separate physician's fee, and agreed rates vary between different parts of the country.

Physicians are paid salaries in public hospitals, and fee-for-service in private hospitals. There are some facilities for private practice within public hospitals, and public hospital doctors are allowed to work in private hospitals (but with some limitations).

Ambulatory care

About 40% of doctors are in general practice and 60% in specialist practice. There are no geographical restrictions on where a doctor may practise. Patients have the choice of consulting either a generalist or a specialist directly. They may seek second or third opinions within the social security system (although, of course needing to meet copayment costs).

The fee-for-service remuneration system gives incentives to GPs to maintain the care of their patients outside hospital, but incentives to specialists to admit patients to private hospitals. Domiciliary nursing care is available on a GPs recommendation from nurses working in independent professional practice, paid fee-for-service by social security.

To overcome the tendency for practitioners to charge higher fees than the nationally negotiated scales, a two-level system of remuneration has been developed. Level 1 is standard. Level 2 fees are paid to 30% of doctors deciding to work at this higher level of service—but requires patients to pay higher social security contributions or special mutuelle or private insurance contributions.

Public health

Public health medicine

Public health is practised at various levels in the French health care system. The Ministry of Health, with regional and department administration (through the prefect) has responsibility for planning and regulating hospitals and independent practitioners. The social security funds have a separate regional and departmental structure, linked to the regional and departmental general councils.

Prevention falls between these two systems. For example, infectious disease control is the responsibility of the Ministry of Health through the local department, whereas child health services are the responsibility of the departmental general council; but both are funded through social security.

Health information is also held at various levels, but is not co-ordinated. Hospital information systems are developing rapidly, but are not population based. The social security funds hold substantial data but do not share them with other bodies. There are regional bodies co-ordinating information, Organisations Régionaux de la Santé, but these differ widely in their levels of funding and capabilities. Epidemiological data are gained as much from primary surveys as from secondary information systems.

Undergraduate teaching

Most universities have established social medicine departments with a range of statistics, health economics and epidemiology research and teaching.

Postgraduate training

There are several paths for training in public health. In the fifth of the seven years of undergraduate medical training, students can choose a specialty (including general practice). They may enrol with the faculty of that specialty within the university and then spend at least four years attached to the faculty. The specialty training includes four terms of clinical practice, of which (for public health) one must be outside a hospital (but not necessarily in public health work).

Further university courses, leading to a diploma, give more specialised public health training. The French School of Public Health at Rennes trains professional staff to work within the Ministry of Health, at central, regional or local level. The social security bodies, also at national, regional and local level, have some doctors working within them; some of these have clinical responsibilities for reviewing sickness claims.

Public health remains an unattractive specialty for doctors in France, partly because there are few high quality university departments for study, and partly because of the lack of appropriate training and career posts within the health system. Although no single specialty of public health exists, the French Society of Public Health is currently proposing to improve liaison between the existing branches of public health practice and the university departments.

GERMANY

Introduction

Since the unification of Germany in 1990, the population of the country is 78.5 million covering an area of 356,900 sq km. The economy continues to be among the strongest in the EC, but is faced with substantial new problems in the east. There is decentralisation from the federal to the state level. The present government is a coalition of the Christian Democrat, Christian Socialist and Free Democratic Parties.

Health care system

In 1883, Germany was the first country in the world to introduce compulsory social insurance for employees. This required employers to provide income support for employees during sickness, and for certain health care payments: it formed the basis for the compulsory health insurance system that operates today. The health care system of the former West German state is described here.

Health care is among the most regulated sectors of the German economy. Responsibilities are split between federal and state governments. The Ministry of Health is responsible for areas such as communicable disease, drugs and hospital financing. Federal health laws are generally implemented at a state level. Coordination between the two levels of administration is mediated through conferences of federal and state health and social ministries. There are also advisory boards at the state and federal levels.

Central government also provides regulation via a number of other ministries. The Ministry of Youth, Family Affairs, Women and Health plays a major role covering drugs and health professionals. The Ministry of Labour and Social Affairs covers hospitals, statutory health insurance, rehabilitation and doctors' fees. The environment, research and technology are also each covered by separate ministries.

Finance

National health insurance is compulsory for all wage-earners, except 10% of people with high incomes. The insurance covers dependents and is also extended to pensioners, students, the armed forces, people with disabilities and people registered unemployed. About 6% of high income earners are voluntary members and most of the rest have private insurance. Only 0.03% of the population remain uninsured.

There are seven major health insurance funds, comprising some 1,300 local sickness funds. General health insurance funds cover seamen, farmers, miners, and those belonging to large companies, while special funds cover groups of workers such as technicians. All funds are obliged to have equal benefits and equal non risk-related premiums. However, there is some competition between them in areas such as sick pay, counselling and spa reimbursements. Special health funds can advertise while general funds cannot. Over the past 20 years there has been a shift towards membership of special funds, and they now have 21% of the market while general funds have 45%. Nevertheless, people generally cannot exercise much choice over which fund they belong to, and the local insurance fund must accept anyone not covered by other funds.

Contributions by the workforce are shared equally between the employee and the employer and average (with wide variations) 12% of total income. The sickness funds reimburse the providers directly. The patient presents the doctor with a voucher which is then submitted quarterly by the doctor to the Association of Health Insurance Doctors.

Approximately 8% of people covered by statutory sickness insurance have supplementary private insurance, which allows more choice of physicians and better facilities. Otherwise, private health insurance is mainly for those who are self-employed or in the highest income brackets. Private premiums are age, sex and risk-related and only cover the primary policy holder. Dependants need their own policy. There is a considerable variety in the extent of coverage available but all policies must give lifelong protection. Since premiums are risk-related, those who are high-risk are more likely to opt for voluntary membership of the national insurance system as it will be less expensive. People covered by private insurance must pay for services directly and then seek reimbursement.

Providers of health care

Hospitals

In the acute sector, 54% of hospitals are public, state or municipal, 42% are charitable non-profit, mainly church and Red Cross, and

4% private for-profit. Hospitals are reimbursed on daily costs by payments from the sickness funds and the private health insurance companies. The amount paid varies by state agreement, with a minimum determined federally. Daily payments thus differ between hospitals but are the same for each patient in any particular hospital. Past cost data are used to calculate the daily rate which is paid to the hospital as a prospective budget.

Hospital building is regulated by the federal government as there is an excess of hospital beds. The capital expenditure for hospitals comes from state taxation. Many tests are either repeated, or carried out in hospital, because ambulatory care doctors often do not have access to hospital facilities. In addition, hospitals, with the exception of university hospitals, do not have outpatient departments. Lack of long-stay facilities leads some acute hospital beds to be filled inappropriately.

Hospital doctors are paid salaries based on the daily rates. Generally they are not allowed to undertake ambulatory care. A small proportion of specialists, for example in ENT and ophthalmology, are office-based with admitting rights.

Ambulatory care

In 1985, 45% of all doctors were office based and 60% of these were specialists. There is competition between specialists and GPs, as specialists can prescribe procedures such as ECGs and X-rays. There is also competition because of the increasing number of doctors practising in the country.

Most ambulatory care doctors practise privately, whether they are GPs or specialists. There is an increasing tendency toward group practices, although there remain significant numbers of single-handed practitioners. Patients can choose any doctor on the panel of their insurance organisation and are relatively free to change them.

The majority of ambulatory care doctors are members of one of the 18 insurance doctors' associations. These bodies negotiate with health insurance funds at state and federal levels to determine doctors' pay. Remuneration is on an item-of-service basis: there are over 4,000 items on the fee schedules. A lump sum is paid to the insurance doctors' associations which is then shared out under a prospective budget system. If payments go over the agreed budget then there is an overall deflator, ie a percentage drop in each doctor's salary to ensure that there is adherence to the budget.

Private insurance companies also have a fixed range for item-of-service payments.

Home nursing and other social services are provided by over 3,800 voluntary organisations. Payment for these services is covered by the sickness funds, although some services require a doctor's certificate for reimbursement.

Public health

Public health services are under local state government control and are financed from local taxes. Every administrative district has a health office in which there is a medical officer and a variety of other workers such as nurses, sanitary engineers and dentists.

Public health medicine

Public health doctors have responsibility for environmental hazards and communicable disease control, some aspects of psychiatric services, and hospital and food hygiene. Other traditional functions, including maternal and child health, preventive medicine and health education have been taken over by GPs and specialists and are paid through insurance reimbursement. There are also proposals for school and young people's medicine to be transferred to paediatricians in private practice.

Undergraduate teaching

Social medicine is compulsory in medical school and is taught in the fourth or fifth years. Epidemiology is not well established, and teaching may be covered by medical sociologists and occupational health physicians.

Postgraduate training

There is a branch of medicine identified as the specialty of medical officers of health. Schools of public health in Düsseldorf and Munich run specialist courses for both doctors and non-doctors, with an examination set at the end. However, the future of public health doctors in Germany is not clear at present. Unsuccessful attempts have been made to define and co-ordinate training programmes but there is no formal training for epidemiologists, with the exception of some summer courses. Health services research, in association with the sickness funds, is now developing.

GREECE

Introduction

Greece is a country of approximately 9.9 million people, with a surface area of 132,000 sq km. More than 3 million live in Athens, while much of the rest of the population is dispersed in rural towns and villages. The terrain is mountainous, and there are also many small islands, so that there are difficulties in access.

Greece has passed through several periods of political change during the twentieth century, with the last period of military dictatorship from 1967–1974. Greece joined the European Community in 1982. The economy shows slow growth, and there is a large government financial deficit due to the combination of increasing expenditure on services, low taxes (income tax is half the European average) and widespread tax evasion.

Health care system

The Greek health care system is currently in transition from a fragmented mixed public and private health system towards a national health service. The law creating the National Health Service (NHS) was passed by parliament in 1983, but it has been implemented only in part.

The Ministry of Health has a Central Health Council which advises the government on national strategies for planning and development. The NHS is intended to have regional councils with similar responsibilities, and with devolution of the administration of the health services, but these arrangements have not yet been implemented.

The NHS law has brought public hospitals into a single system under the direction of the Ministry, and established a network of rural health centres staffed by full-time salaried doctors. However, ambulatory care by specialists continues in the larger towns, and has prevented the wide development of general practice.

Greece has one of the highest rates of doctors per head of population in Europe, a further factor in the expansion of specialist ambulatory care.

Finance

The NHS intends to establish a unified single health fund. However, at present there are broadly two health care sectors, hospital and ambulatory care, which are separately financed. There are more than 300 non-profit insurance funds covering about 99% of the population; the two largest, for private sector employees and rural workers, have about 70% coverage between them. Except for rural workers, employers and employees both contribute to the funds.

Public hospitals are financed mainly by the state, with health funds contributing only 10-15% of the total costs. The funds pay for all ambulatory care, except for that from health centres. But they have different methods of providing ambulatory care, either through employing their own staff or through fee-for-service reimbursement with doctors in private practice. Costs per capita, and thus benefits, differ widely between the funds.

Patients are initially expected to seek care within the arrangements defined by their health fund. Thus, private sector employees will go to one of the clinics maintained by their fund, while rural workers will go to one of the government's 1,500 rural health dispensaries (staffed by medical graduates compulsorily in their first year of work). Others will go to a specialist working under fee-for-service contract to the specific fund.

Providers of care

Hospitals

The NHS law sought to diminish private competition and market influences in health care. The state took over most non-private hospitals (eg Red Cross, ecclesiastic, municipal), so that about two-thirds now are public. The hospitals are inappropriately distributed, with half of all beds in the greater Athens region, and many have low occupancy.

Doctors working in government hospitals have been expected, since 1985, to work full-time without private practice. While health care is officially free, there is evidence that many hospital doctors charge an undeclared 'copayment' directly to patients, both in hospital and ambulatory care, providing a substantial increase in their incomes.

The remaining private hospitals tend to be small, providing surgical or long-stay care. While private hospitals were not formally abolished, there are restrictions on establishing new hospitals and limits on the acceptable size of hospitals. Since there is no public funding for stays in these hospitals and the health funds may only reimburse 10–20% of the costs, there was a steady decline in private hospitals during the 1980s. The new government since 1989, however, has given greater support to private hospitals.

Ambulatory care

The rural dispensaries are mainly staffed by recent graduates undertaking compulsory service. The proposed network of health centres would eventually require about 3,000 GPs, but at present few doctors are trained or seek to work as GPs.

Doctors working in the ambulatory care clinics of insurance funds are salaried but part-time. Otherwise, doctors predominantly work as private specialists, increasingly using ambulatory investigation centres (imaging, pathology, cardiac). While patients may be referred by GPs, direct attendance at specialist clinics in the main towns and at tertiary hospitals provides a wide range of ways for patients to obtain secondary care.

Public health

In the early part of the twentieth century there were substantial developments of public health. A Ministry of Health was established in 1918. Services were developed to combat malaria and dengue, and traditional environmental health services, of water supply and sewage, and maternal and child care, were brought to rural areas; in consequence, infectious diseases declined substantially. However, with better communications, the rural population had access to specialist services in towns and the public health services went into decline. The major new environmental issue for Athens, atmospheric pollution, has become the responsibility of a new Ministry of the Environment.

Public health medicine

Each of the 52 administrative divisions of the country has a public health department with a range of responsibilities: supervision of the dispensaries; payment of the Civil Servants' Health Fund fees to specialists; communicable disease and environmental control; immunisations; health education; and (officially) care for drug dependent and alcoholic patients. While these duties appear extensive, public health departments have poor status and poor recruitment, not least because, without private practice, income is lower than in other fields of medicine.

The NHS law specifies the creation of divisions of social

medicine, which should be equivalent to the four other divisions of medicine, surgery, laboratory and psychiatry. The Central Health Services Council has described social medicine divisions within the NHS to be responsible for:

- applied epidemiology
- environmental health
- prevention of infectious and chronic diseases
- health education promotion
- occupational health
- health services planning and evaluation
- health information systems

The divisions should direct their attention towards the population served by the hospital, and work closely with health centres which provide primary health care to integrate services. They are separate from, but work closely with, the public health departments.

Undergraduate teaching

Public health training for medical students is usually limited to lectures on hygiene, with some introduction to epidemiology. Academic public health departments are not well established in medical schools.

Postgraduate training

Since 1987, four-year training has been required for doctors taking up social medicine: one year general experience, one year academic training at the national School of Public Health in Athens, and two years' practical training. However, in practice either a Diploma in hygiene from the School of Public Health or a PhD from a University is regarded as sufficient for a specialist position. Social medicine is also taught as an undergraduate subject in some medical schools.

IRELAND

Introduction

Ireland, a republic since 1922, has a population of 3.5 million covering an area of 68,895 sq km. It has one of the lower levels of economic development in the Community and a net ouflow of population. Parliamentary politics are affected by the position of Northern Ireland, which remains part of the UK.

Health care system

Health care is provided by a complex mixture of privately and publicly organised services. Under the Department of Health, eight regional health boards are responsible for populations varying in size from 200,000 to a million people. The boards administer all aspects of health care and also some social services. Each board is organised into sectors for hospital and community services, and in some boards there is also a sector for the specialist hospitals. The health boards have a membership of local authority representatives, professionals and a small number of ministerial appointments.

The Department of Health provides public funding for the regional health boards. It also has some direct control over public hospitals in areas such as changes in the numbers of facilities or the siting of high technology services.

Finance

The state is estimated to pay about 80% of health care costs, most spending being on the hospital sector. The public system is directly financed, but there is also significant funding and subsidy of the private sector. Health insurance premiums are tax deductible, but this is being reconsidered.

There are two categories of eligibility for tax-financed health care:

Category 1 (the 'General Medical Service' (GMS)), covering 38% of the population, is for low-income families and dependants, the elderly on social welfare or dependants of a person working in an EC member state. GMS patients are entitled to all standard services, which excludes private or semi-private accommodation or services from a GP other than the one with whom they are registered. These services are free.

Category 2, covering most of the rest of the population, has eligibility determined by personal income. In theory, it should cover middle-income groups, but exceptions occur as dependants and other wage earners are not taken into account. Category 2 patients are able to use public wards and specialist outpatient clinics, and receive some dental, optician and audiological services. GP care and drugs are not included. Health insurance for category 2 patients is virtually all provided by the Voluntary Health Insurance Board (VHI). VHI is a state-run non-profit organisation set up in 1957. The board is appointed by the Ministry of Health. The premiums charged are based on broad ratings and not adjusted for individual risk factors. Of the two schemes provided, over 90% of people choose the broader package including payment for private facilities. VHI's monopoly position allows it to negotiate with the hospitals and professionals. It also has some freedom to fix its own prices for its customers.

Providers of health care

Hospitals

Hospitals can be public, private not-for-profit or private for-profit. Public hospitals, including some acute hospitals and many of the psychiatric hospitals, are owned and run by the health boards. The state also funds the voluntary public hospitals which are privately owned, often by religious orders, and provide much of the acute care. Most of the teaching hospitals fall into this group. The Department of Health provides up to 90% of the running costs for these voluntary hospitals, but has little control over how the money is spent. Their income is gained from private beds covered by VHI. The private for-profit hospital sector which charges fees directly to patients is expanding and owns about 9% of beds.

All doctors must choose one of the three contracts, either all salaried public work, all private fee-for-service work, or a mixture. Doctors are entitled to use hospital facilities for private work if they have the correct contract, and no charges are then made to the doctor by the hospital. This has led to suggestions of a double standard in care—shorter waiting times and better facilities appear to be available to those who pay.

Ambulatory care

GPs are self-employed independent professionals. They may set up practice in any area of their choice. The majority work as single-handed practitioners. They are paid by capitation for category 1 patients by the health boards but, as VHI does not provide cover for GP care, much of their income is derived from direct fee-for-service charges. There is no fixed price scale for these services.

Public health

Public health is located within the community care sector of the health boards. This has led to some problems as it gives practitioners in the area little opening into the hospital sector. Recently, a working party reported to the Minister of Health to suggest that public health should be incorporated into the board level of administration. This would give public health a broader remit for action.

Public health medicine

Public health medicine was recognised as a specialty in 1979, although there is no formal register of practitioners as yet. Doctors within the specialty may work within a broad spectrum of areas from environmental hazard and communicable disease control to service planning and evaluation. The majority work as senior clinical medical officers.

Undergraduate teaching

Public health forms part of the undergraduate curriculum in all five medical schools. Two schools provide introductory pre-clinical courses and all teach a course in the clinical years which is both compulsory and examined.

Postgraduate training

Training in public health is organised by the Faculty of Public Health Medicine. A specialist training of three years post-internship in a variety of clinical posts leads to taking the written Part 1 Membership examination of the Faculty. Higher specialist training, entered through competitive interview, includes three years in an approved post attached to a senior public health doctor and one year in a senior post. A Part II examination, consisting of a written thesis and an oral examination, is taken during the final years of training. The training is common for public health doctors and academic epidemiologists.

ITALY

Introduction

Italy is a long peninsula stretching from the Alps south to the Mediterranean, with a wide range of climates and strong regional traditions. The country has 57 million inhabitants and covers 301,200 sq km. United as one country in 1870, Italy became a republic (by referendum) in 1945. Since this time, one major political party has held power within a series of coalition governments, and rapid development has brought Italy among the leading world economies.

Devolution of some government responsibilities to regions (19 regions and two autonomous provinces) in the early 1970s was a spur to the integration of hospitals, and subsequently of general practice, within the public sector. Regions now hold the main political power in the development of health services. The lower tier of government, the communes, are far too varied in size to manage the services effectively—the 8,000 communes ranging from cities of several million to rural communities of less than a thousand. Long-standing differences in cultures between the northern, central and southern regions lead to significant variations in health services.

Health care system

Most health care in Italy is provided through the National Health Service (NHS), but some is private. There are three levels of care: GP, polyclinic and hospital. Health services are regulated by a pyramidal structure, from central Ministry to regions to local health units.

The NHS was established in 1980. It assures comprehensive health services to all citizens through GPs, and specialist care by polyclinic or hospital outpatient consultation or by hospital admission. The range of local NHS services includes mental health care, occupational health, veterinary services and family planning, but the extent of provision is determined locally.

The NHS is funded through central government and distributed through regions and (currently) 670 local health units (LHUs). The regions are politically elected bodies, with a range of functions of which health care is the largest. LHUs are bodies with members appointed by local political bodies (communes). They manage the

GP contracts, and the polyclinic and hospital services, within a defined resident population (mostly in the range 50,000 to 200,000).

Although nationally the system is uniform, locally it is markedly varied in its implementation: in general, the services in the north and centre of Italy are better than in the south. This is partly due to different levels of finance, partly to differences in economic development and partly to political factors.

While Italy has the largest number of graduate doctors in any EC country due to open registration in the universities during the 1970s and 1980s, the limits on hospital and GP practice have led to many under-employed and unemployed doctors. Some are employed by the NHS to provide out-of-hours emergency cover for GPs, others work without pay in hospitals and clinics.

Finance

Finance for the NHS is raised through compulsory national health insurance augmented by support from national taxes.

Health insurance is deducted directly from salaries or contributed to the government by self-employed people. A fixed proportion of salary is paid, currently around 12% for employed people, up to a maximum upper limit of income. For salaried workers, almost all the contribution is made by the employer. For self-employed workers the contribution is lower. All citizens must use the public insurance system, and they receive the same benefits.

There are copayments for drugs, ambulatory dental care, and some prostheses, with exemption for low-income patients. Most dental care is paid privately. A variety of different copayment systems and levels has been tried, but they contribute only a small proportion of total health spending. An attempt by the government in the late 1980s to introduce copayments for hospital outpatient attendances and inpatient stays was defeated.

The government contributes to the NHS total in two ways: first, as a defined contribution to the NHS budget of up to about 30% at the start of the fiscal year; and second, in filling the gap at the end of the year between the set budget and the true spending. Setting a budget below the projected spend has been seen as a device for containing costs, but the division between the centre which raises the money through taxes and the regions which spend the money has not led to satisfactory control.

The private health insurance market is small, covering probably less than 5% of the population. It is mainly paid by employers and can provide a 'top up' cost to allow an employee to receive private rather than public care.

The NHS budget is distributed each year according to a formula that seeks to redress the historic imbalance in spending between regions: some success was achieved in equity during the 1980s. However, larger differences in per capita spending exist within regions, mainly because of clustering of hospitals in larger towns. The regions allocate their budgets by LHU within sub-headings of hospitals, GPs, public health, etc. The lack of general hospitals in up to a quarter of LHUs has been one of the spurs towards recent proposals to amalgamate LHUs into larger units of population.

Providers of care

Hospitals

Most hospitals are owned by the regions within the NHS. There are, however, contracts between the state and some prestigious independent hospitals, including research and church-owned hospitals. These receive special funding. There are around 600 private hospitals, including some for-profit hospitals, but these are mainly small and not usually owned by multinational health care companies. Private hospitals mainly depend on NHS payments for their income; patients are able to 'top up' the NHS contribution to the level charged by the private hospital. In national surveys the public appears to consider that private hospitals are cleaner and more comfortable, but medical care is regarded as better in public hospitals. There is no perceived difference in the standard of food.

Doctors working in public hospitals may be full or part-time (at all grades); there are about equal numbers of each. They are paid a salary. Officially, full-time doctors should not undertake private practice.

Ambulatory care

Citizens are registered with a GP in the commune where they officially reside (there is compulsory national registration of residence). GPs should have list sizes of 500 to 1,500. Children under 12 should be cared for separately by paediatrician GPs. GPs are paid by capitation: there are no fees for individual services.

Referral for ambulatory specialist referral may be to an NHS polyclinic, to a private specialist or to a hospital outpatient consultation. Private specialists are more common in the south of the country. Consultations must be by GP referral, and the LHU must agree the referral if it is to be paid for by the NHS: thus patients experience a rather cumbersome bureaucracy. Polyclinic doctors are paid sessional rates for a fixed number of consultations; private specialists charge a fee-for-service to the NHS.

There is a lack of community-based nursing within the NHS, but private, usually church, organisations provide some non-professional domiciliary services. One special feature of the Italian NHS in the 1980s has been the move towards community psychiatric care. Many reports confirm that this has been highly successful where it has been initiated by medical staff and supported by the LHU and commune, but has failed where psychiatrists are uninterested and investment in local facilities has been inadequate.

Public health

Public health medicine

Provincial NHS hygiene departments are responsible for monitoring environmental health, including ensuring that services keep within environmental health laws, while laboratories undertake analyses and are responsible for communicable disease control. Each region is required, by the NHS law, to establish an 'epidemiological observatory' to determine health needs and assist in planning. In some regions these observatories have been well funded and have made important contributions. The NHS structure has opportunities for public health medicine also at LHU level: expansion will depend partly on the development of appropriate training. The Italian Society for Hygiene and Public Health is committed to developing accreditation for public health schools and teaching programmes, but there is no formally recognised specialist 'professional board' within or outside the main medical union.

Undergraduate teaching

Communicable disease control and hygiene are taught in all medical schools; epidemiology, including statistics and epidemiological methods, is more often voluntary and depends on available staff. The universities have substantial autonomy in deciding their curricula.

Postgraduate training

Doctors can specialise at any stage after graduation without any formal clinical experience. Given the lack of opportunities for clinical practice for recent graduates, there is an incentive towards specialisation: over 100 different specialties are recognised. Universities offer four-year training courses in public health, with specialisation in hygiene, district service planning or hospital administration. There is no co-ordination of standards between courses. Doctors working for five years in a specialist post, whether or not they have been formally trained, are automatically recognised as a specialist by law.

Epidemiological research is developing strongly in the universities, regional departments and local health units.

LUXEMBOURG

Introduction

Luxembourg is the smallest member state in the European Community. It has a population of 370,000 in a country that covers 2,586 sq km. It is a wealthy country, dependent on a declining steel industry and a rapidly expanding financial sector. Government is by proportional representation, with usually a coalition of the Christian and Social Democratic Parties.

Health care system

Compulsory health insurance covers almost all the population and is part of the social security system. As the country is small there is little decentralisation of administration. The Ministry of Health has responsibility for areas such as hospital planning and the purchase of certain medical equipment. The planning of new hospitals must take account of local and national need. This is determined by analysis of the 'health chart' of the country, a collection of relevant service information. The organisation of hospital services takes place at three regional levels.

Finance

The 12 sickness funds have membership based on social and occupational groups. Membership is compulsory and there is no choice over the fund to which an individual belongs. Premiums are fixed by law as a percentage of gross earnings up to a maximum of five times the legal minimum wage. Contributions are shared equally between employer and employee. For workers who are self-employed, farmers, or others who are voluntarily insured, the whole contribution is payable by the individual.

Cover includes medical and dental services, travelling costs and pharmaceuticals. There is copayment for drugs usually with 80% reimbursement. Patients are also expected to contribute to inpatient care at a set rate per day. Patients have completely free choice over the doctor and hospital that care for them. As all doctors automatically work for the social security system, this gives extensive choice.

The state covers the contributions for certain groups of people:

students, school pupils, invalids. In addition, it covers areas such as maternity care, road traffic accidents if there is no third party insurance cover, and school sports accidents. The state also provides free care for high-risk groups needing care for more than three months, including patients with tuberculosis, polio, mental illness and cancers.

Private insurance offers only a very limited contribution to health care, for example some increase in comfort or coverage of treatment abroad.

Providers of care

Hospitals

Almost all hospitals are not-for-profit, divided between private ownership, mainly by religious institutions, and ownership by the local communes. There is one for-profit hospital in the country. Hospitals are classified as acute, long- or medium-stay according to their degrees of specialisation. Payment to the hospitals is made by the health funds at rates agreed by the hospitals and representatives of the social security system.

Doctors are paid a fee for service which is agreed between their professional organisations and social security. Doctors are free to work where they like and many have their own practice as well as working in the hospitals.

Ambulatory care

Both GPs and specialists work in the community, with patients having free access to either. They are all paid by item of service. Fees are negotiated nationally, and all doctors are obliged to abide by them. Specialists outnumber GPs more than two to one. There are very few health centres, and most practitioners work alone. However, some hospitals are setting up polyclinics.

The Red Cross runs a system of child health clinics that oversee the development of the under-two-year-olds. The communes are responsible for the school health services provided by local GPs.

Public health

There is no comprehensively organised public health system. The Ministry of Health is responsible for the quality of drinking water. The National Institute for Hygiene and Public Health is attached to the Ministry and is responsible for laboratory services for toxicology and microbiology as well as determining standards for food. Public health medicine is not identified as a specialty in the country, and there are no academic departments of public health or epidemiology.

NETHERLANDS

Introduction

The Netherlands has a population of 14.9 million and covers an area of 33,937 sq km. This makes the country one of the most densely populated in Europe. The Netherlands is a constitutional monarchy and parliamentary democracy. The country has 12 provinces and 714 municipalities. There is significant decentralisation of government responsibility for areas such as health, transport and education.

Health care system

The main body for central control is the Ministry of Welfare, Health and Cultural Affairs. There is decentralisation of administration to the provinces and some of the major towns. Generally provinces are responsible for inpatient care and regional health plans, which require central ministerial approval. Municipalities are responsible for community care including environmental health, school health and health education.

Whilst central government has played a key part in planning, it is hoped that introducing managed competition will lessen this role. Central government will then focus on legislation and regulation, including anti-cartel policing, quality control and information disclosure. At present there is a surplus both of beds and of doctors in the country. It is hoped that the new system will address this problem.

The insurance system is overseen centrally by the Health Insurance Funds Council. The State Inspectorate of Health has a role independent of the Ministry, although it is responsible to it, and ensures that certain statutory regulations, eg for food safety, are observed.

Finance

Statutory insurance for 'exceptional' medical expenses, covering hospital stays of more than one year, all psychiatric care, readmissions within a year, nursing homes, vaccinations and a variety of other social and long-term medical services, is compulsory for the working population. Contributions are split between the employer and employee, with the self-employed paying the whole premium. People over 65 and under 15 do not pay contributions.

For other health care, there are broadly three groups of insurance: (i) approximately 65% of the population is covered statutorily by the state scheme, with contributions from both employers and employees. This group includes employees earning below a fixed wage level, their families and those in receipt of social security; (ii) five per cent of the population who are government employees, such as civil servants and teachers, are covered by their own special schemes; (iii) about 30% of the population has private insurance.

The majority of other medical care, including industrial injury and disease, is covered by individual personal insurance. Most care is free at the point of use, with copayment for some dentistry, some maternity care and transport other than ambulance. Ninety per cent of people take out supplementary cover, especially for maternity care which has a tradition of independent practice.

Within the state insurance scheme people are obliged to join a fund within their geographical area. Some occupational groups such as seamen have their own particular fund. With the implementation of the reforms, increasing competition may be brought about by allowing people to join any fund.

Private insurance premiums are risk-related and only cover the policy holder. Premiums are not related to income. Children are charged at 50% the adult rate. In 1986 the government legislated that all insurers should provide a standard cover package. This provides insurance for the elderly, who no longer have a separate scheme. It also covers others who used to be insured under the abolished voluntary insurance scheme. Standard cover is not age or risk-related. Ultimately, insurers will be compensated by receiving a risk-related grant from a central body that collects all income-related premiums. The flat-rate premium will be paid direct to the insurers.

Providers of health care

Hospitals

Most of the 190 acute hospitals are general, with a few specialised institutions. For-profit hospitals are illegal, and the majority are privately owned, usually by church-related organisations. Seven of the eight teaching hospitals are state owned.

Hospitals are paid by the insurance companies on a prospective budget system based on historical cost data. Payments are made for each day of stay, and a weighted average is used rather than an actual cost. There is a state subsidy for teaching hospitals and some services such as transplants, abortion services and research. Government subsidies are also given for public health services such as school health, environmental hazard protection and tuberculosis prevention.

Hospital doctors are specialists and a GP must refer a patient in order to be seen by a specialist. They are paid by item of service, and the majority contract their services and pay rent to the hospital. A few are salaried. Most specialists work in partnerships and provide outpatient as well as inpatient care.

Primary care

GPs are predominantly single-handed private practitioners: few work from health centres. They are paid a capitation fee for two-thirds of their patients and additional fee-for-service payments. The capitation payments cover those patients who have statutory insurance. Payments are made by the sickness funds and private insurers. The latter are being encouraged to provide coverage for primary care to help prevent the specialist being the first point of contact for some patients (as these consultations will be paid for). Up to the present, any GP who wanted to contract with the insurers could do so. The new system will allow insurers to choose which providers they work with. GPs require the permission of the municipalities to practise in any given area.

Professional home care, especially home nurses, is organised by the National Cross Organisations and financed under the Exceptional Medical Expenses Act. Recently, there has been a significant increase in the number of private organisations that provide this type of care.

Public health

Public health is mainly decentralised, with central inspectorates for food and environmental protection. Much of the organised prevention—vaccination and cervical smear tests, for example—is carried out by municipalities, as is environmental health. Within municipal health services and other departments of public health non-medical staff may carry out public health functions.

Public health medicine

The specialty that is nearest to the British concept of public health medicine is termed 'general health care', a sub-specialty of social medicine. There are about 250 practitioners registered throughout the country. Occupational health, youth health care and insurance medicine are the other branches of this specialty. Within general health care doctors can have diverse areas of practice, including administrative/policy positions in government or as hospital directors or in preventive health care in municipal health services. Specialists in communicable diseases tend to be found only in larger towns.

Undergraduate teaching

All medical schools run courses in social medicine. These courses are based on lectures, seminars and clerkships. There is no standardisation of what should be taught. There may also be courses in statistics, sociology and epidemiology.

Postgraduate training

After registration, a doctor can choose to train in social medicine through part-time courses organised by private institutions such as the institutes in Leiden and Utrecht. The courses are usually paid for by employers and there is little state subsidy. The courses cover areas such as basic epidemiology, economics, interpersonal skills and organisational issues in health care. Statistics and sociology tend not to be taught in as much depth. The emphasis is on applied, rather than research or evaluation orientated, skills. In order to pass the course, attendance records and various library-based submissions are required. There are no examinations. These courses are open to both medical and non-medical students. However, only doctors can be registered in the specialty. Registration is not automatically required for employment although it increases the chances of getting a job.

New plans to create a National School of Public Health are being developed for 1992. This will provide two MSc courses, one in epidemiology and one in community health. The courses will be split between two universities. It is proposed that there should be two levels of qualifications, at MSc and PhD level. Health services research is carried out in a number of organisations: some private firms offer the service, as do some university departments and medical schools and some non-university agencies.

PORTUGAL

Introduction

Portugal is a republic of 9.81 million people, and covers an area of 92,100 sq km. It has had territorial identity for 800 years and significant colonial links, especially with Brazil (independent in the nineteenth century) and Mozambique and Angola (independent in 1975). In the post-war period, Portugal was ruled by dictatorship and industrialisation was slower than in other EC countries. Democratic government was re-established in 1974, and Portugal entered the EC in 1986. While economic progress in the last decade has been substantial, there remain large social inequalities: for example, the illiteracy rate is estimated at 18%, although now mostly in older people.

Health care system

The health care system in Portugal reflects three periods of progress and reform. Until the 1970s, health care was traditional and provided in the larger cities and towns, with private medical practice for the rich, ambulatory polyclinics for insured people, and public hospitals, often founded and managed by the Catholic Church, for the poor. From 1971 there was a rapid development of health care provided publicly in health centres, led by growing numbers of public health trained physicians.

A national health service reform in 1979 brought together the different historical elements of health care, with a structure controlled by the Ministry of Health and devolved through local administrative bodies. While about 80% of health care is provided within the public sector, there are significant contributions from charitable bodies and for-profit private clinics.

Finance

Three different forms of finance contribute to health care in Portugal. The National Health Service (NHS) is financed through public taxes, and is available to the whole population through health centres and public hospitals. However, some sectors of public service and large private companies retain insurance based fee-for-service care for their staff. A small proportion of the population also retain their own health insurance, which has some incentive through tax exemptions.

Because of the use of private ambulatory specialists (mainly radiology and laboratory medicine), about one-third of public health care spending is transferred to private providers.

Portugal spends well under the EC average on health care although, in contrast to most other EC countries, more is spent on primary health care than on hospitals. To increase finance, the better off would need either to pay for more health insurance or pay more taxes. A wider spread of income through industrialisation is likely to be the solution to better provision.

Providers of health care

Hospitals

Hospital doctors working in the public sector are all salaried. The large majority of hospitals are public, integrated into a network of district, central and university hospitals. The hospitals serve specified catchment areas, and are able to refer 'up' the hierarchy for more specialised care. Hospitals receive their finance directly from the Ministry of Health.

Private hospitals include those run by religious organisations and a small number of private for-profit hospitals. The medical staff are usually salaried staff from the public hospital who are paid a fee-for-service when working in the private hospitals.

Ambulatory care

The two forms of public ambulatory care—the traditional insurance polyclinics and government health centres—were integrated by the NHS, and are controlled by district health administrations. The integrated health centres include GPs and public health doctors, nurses, social workers and some specialists. They provide some preventive care, for example maternal and child health, but their orientation is increasingly towards treatment. The health centres have allowed the majority of medical graduates in the 1980s to enter general practice, and postgraduate training courses have been established.

Substantial use is made by the public sector of the private sector for investigations, and this has limited growth of the public sector in this field.

Public health

Public health doctors were strongly represented in the health service reforms of the 1970s, and the health centres were planned to serve defined populations.

Public health medicine

A College of Public Health Medicine has been established within the Portuguese Medical Association. Public health is seen broadly to include communicable disease control and environmental health; health promotion and prevention; health services planning and policies; and academic research. However, merger of the health centres run directly by the public health service into the integrated NHS health centres providing both prevention and treatment has lessened the priority attached to public health. New forms of practice, working within the NHS at several levels, are now developing.

Undergraduate teaching

The five medical schools have similar curricula, with social sciences and statistics in the first year, epidemiology in the third year and public health in the final (sixth) year.

Postgraduate training

Specialist training is controlled nationally and regionally through competitive entry into NHS training posts. Appointments are for three years, with the second academic year at the National School of Public Health in Lisbon. New masters degrees in epidemiology and occupational health are being developed by other universities to complement training at the National School.

SPAIN

Introduction

Spain is a country of 39 million inhabitants occupying an area of 504,800 sq km. The country is divided into 17 autonomous regions. State control over many activities has gradually transferred to these regions since the enacting of the Constitution two years after General Franco's death in 1975. Each region has a government council and a legislative assembly. The country is a democracy with a constitutional monarchy.

Health care system

Spain has a national health service funded through general taxation and contributions from insurance premiums. It entitles over 95% of the population to comprehensive coverage. It is supplemented by a complex mix of public and private provision and funding. The main central administrative body for health insurance is the National Institute for Health (INSALUD).

Administrative structures are governed by the General Health Act of 1986. Each region is responsible for the provision of health care for its population. Hospitals and health centres previously run by the state were transferred to the regions, along with most of the staff.

The Ministry of Health and Consumer Affairs in Madrid has retained a role in pharmaceutical legislation, general policy formulation and co-ordination. Central control also exists over the building of health care facilities and quality control of health centres. In addition, the Ministry of Health determines the overall health budget. The budgets allocated to regions have been the subject of considerable controversy and are at present based on the number registered by the social security system. The regions cannot increase or decrease their health budget by intraregional transfer of funds.

Co-ordination occurs via a number of interministerial committees with regional and state representatives. They are responsible for aspects of administration such as allocation of resources. There is also a permanent council that co-ordinates purchasing of certain drugs and has a planning and co-ordinating role.

Regions have health councils that act as advisory bodies and are composed of professionals, users, managers and trades unions.

Direct management is at the level of health areas, each comprising a population of about 200,000. Beneath areas are 'basic health zones' on which primary health care is structured.

Regions are responsible for all aspects of health care including screening programmes and health education. Provincial and municipal areas still hold responsibilities for some welfare and environmental health issues, eg drinking water, vaccinations, the care of psychiatric patients and for those without social security coverage.

Decentralisation has been implemented very variably across the country. Generally, the transfer of non-hospital services has been more successful than acute care. Central responsibility continues for the management of primary care in two regions and of hospital care in all regions.

Finance

The social security system (INSALUD) is financed from two sources: first, by a state contribution from general taxes, and second, by contributions from employers and employees (26% of total earnings from the employer, and 5% from the employee). In 1989 the funding of INSALUD was changed so that now 66% of its money comes from general taxation, 30% from contributions and 4% from other sources. Overall about 80% of health expenditure is financed publicly, of which over half comes from INSALUD, about 12% from local government and the rest from other central government bodies. The 20% from private households is split between direct payments (about 88%) and insurance premiums.

Coverage by the national insurance system is fairly comprehensive. However, mental health services, fertility programmes and plastic surgery are not covered; neither is dental treatment (with the exception of extractions) nor appliances such as glasses and crutches. Only prescription drugs have copayment: 40% of most drugs are paid for by the patient, with the exception of pensioners who receive free treatment, including drugs.

There is a significant private insurance market. Government figures suggest that 161 companies were operating in 1987. However, there has been less growth in the area than expected. It has mainly been composed of mergers, with a few new companies entering the market. There has been difficulty in the private sector in recent years as management has been lacking and some companies have been too small to survive in the world of high-cost medicine.

Estimates suggest that around 24% of households have private insurance, usually in addition to their national insurance. This percentage varies considerably across regions—it is over 30% in Catalonia. The types of packages available are varied, some covering all services and others just specialists' visits. Premiums can be fixed freely by the companies and reflect individual risk factors. About half of private expenditure is on areas not covered by national health insurance, and the rest on direct payments from visits, nursing care and tests, particularly X-rays. Only 2.5% of direct payments are for hospital services.

Providers of health care

Hospitals

The hospital sector is mixed, with publicly owned hospitals (67%) and both for-profit and not-for-profit private hospitals (33%); these percentages are reversed in some regions such as Catalonia. Many of the non-profit hospitals belong to the Church or Red Cross. Public hospitals can belong to the regions, INSALUD, or municipal governments. Generally, the largest (over 500 beds) and most sophisticated hospitals are within the public sector. Many of the private hospitals have only between 20 and 100 beds. However, as the public hospital sector is too small, significant amounts of work are contracted out to the private sector.

Nationally, there are 22 categories of private hospitals, coded according to their facilities. (Some regions have simplified this system: Catalonia, for example, has just three hospital groups.) This coding is then reflected in the payment they receive for working with the national health system. Payment depends on daily costs and numbers of beds.

The private sector can be contracted into the health service only if it is not possible to provide care within the public system and if there are sufficient funds available. Preference is given to the non-profit hospitals. These hospitals can choose to join the national health system so that they are funded publicly, although their ownership remains private. This gives the health authority the ability to regulate their activities. Other private hospitals that are not integrated into the national system can also contract to it, providing that they pass certain quality standards.

Hospital doctors working within the publicly owned system are salaried. Specialists are assigned to one of three groups: hospital, consulting office or home visit. Private specialists are paid a fee for service.

Ambulatory care

Primary health care is undergoing reform with the intention of strengthening the non-hospital sector. 'Basic health zones' are being established. Under these, GPs, paediatricians, social workers, nurses and dentists work together in health centres. They are responsible for a defined geographical area and are expected to provide comprehensive care. They replace the old system whereby GPs worked for two hours a day in clinics and had to visit their patients at home the rest of the time. However, the establishment of health centres has been slow.

All health professionals have the right to practise where they choose, with the exception of working in villages of less than 6,000 inhabitants. Prices and advertising are also not under any restrictions. All patients have a GP whom they can change, but only in limited circumstances. The GP is the first point of contact for health care and can refer to a clinic specialist, the hospital outpatient department or directly to the hospital for admission.

Before the national health service, GPs and ambulatory care specialists were paid by capitation based on the numbers of cards the doctor held. Each card represented a family. Specialists continue with this system: each group has a maximum number of cards for their lists; for example, an endocrinologist is allowed 50,000 whereas surgeons are only allowed 12,000. However, the new system pays primary health care workers a salary which is weighted according to demographic factors.

Public health

Since decentralisation, public health has largely passed to the regional and municipal levels, but with the incomplete transfer of medical care services, problems with co-ordination have resulted. There are significant differences between regions in carrying out prevention functions such as screening programmes.

Public health medicine

The specialty is recognised within medicine as 'preventive medicine and public health'. Doctors within the specialty may be attached to administrative bodies or to hospital preventive medicine departments—more often the latter. These departments have fairly limited functions related to areas such as the occupational health of hospital workers and infection control. There is a faculty for the specialty that is responsible for the content, accreditation and evaluation of training.

Undergraduate teaching

All medical schools are obliged to teach at least 30 hours of public health, usually in the fifth year. Subjects taught include epidemiology, statistics and communicable disease. Sociology, economics and management studies are less widely taught.

Postgraduate training

After the intern year any medical graduate can enter the specialty. Formal training requires an initial academic year followed by a two-year service training. The academic year can be an MSc offered at one of the schools of public health (Madrid, Valencia, Granada, Barcelona) or a health officer's qualification offered by the Madrid National School of Public Health (this is separate from the regional school at Madrid as it is not a university and is run by the Ministry of Health). Health administrators, who are also civil servants, must take a separate administrative examination.

Subsequently, doctors may be attached to preventive medicine or administrative departments for two years. The content of the training during these two years has been stipulated but largely not implemented. In theory, recognition of specialist training can then be applied for from the Minister of Education, if accompanied by a report from the Faculty of Public Health. However, many people have been accepted in substantive posts without this recognition as there has been a shortage of high calibre doctors in the specialty. The approval of posts for training is also not well developed.

There are few academic epidemiologists and the majority are not public health trained. Previously, there were epidemiologists attached to health administration departments, but with reorganisation this role has been eroded. Generally, the links between academic and service departments are not well developed.

UNITED KINGDOM

Introduction

The UK is composed of the countries of England, Wales, Scotland and Northern Ireland, with a population of approximately 56 million and covering 244,786 sq km. The countries are governed by a constitutional monarchy and elected parliament in London. Each constituent country has its own minister and there are differences in legislation and administrative organisation, particularly in Scotland and Northern Ireland.

Health care system

Health care in the UK is provided through the National Health Service (NHS). The position for England is described here, and is broadly the same in the other constituent countries. Health care is free at the point of use and covers the whole resident population. It is funded primarily through general taxation, with a small contribution from insurance. There has been considerable reorganisation of health services since the 1990 National Health Service and Community Care Act was introduced.

The Department of Health is responsible to parliament for financial and managerial control of the NHS, as well as for other duties such as regulation of the pharmaceutical companies, private medicine, nursing homes and health care research. The Department determines the resources given to regional health authorities (health boards in Scotland), covering populations of about three million people. Regions in turn distribute these resources to district health authorities (to purchase hospital and community care) and to family health service authorities (to purchase primary care from GPs, dentists, pharmacists and opticians) according to population, with weightings to take account of demographic and other factors.

The district and family health service authorities are jointly responsible for assessing the needs of, and purchasing services for, their populations ranging in size from 100,000 to over a million people. Services can be contracted from the NHS or from the private sector. Central management of the health service is in the hands of the NHS management executive.

Local authorities, the elected tier of government below parliament, provide housing, social and environmental services as well as education, transport, leisure amenities and town planning. District and family health service authorities and local authorities do not always share the same boundaries, leading to considerable difficulties in joint working and planning.

Finance

National health insurance is levied on all employed people and contributes about 10% of the cost of the NHS. Employers pay an equal share of this contribution. The rest of the funding for the NHS comes from general taxation, with about 4% coming from direct charges such as prescriptions.

The care provided by the NHS is comprehensive and mostly free. However, there is substantial copayment for ambulatory dental treatment, with exemptions for certain groups, such as pregnant women, children and those on income support. There is also a flat rate copayment for drugs and appliances, again with exemptions. Recently, the government has introduced charges for eyesight and hearing tests and has limited NHS glasses to exempted groups only.

Local authority services are paid for by local taxes combined with block grants from central government. The local taxes vary, depending on the size of the central government support grant received and the needs of the local population.

Private medicine in the UK is a small but growing sector. Everybody has the option of taking out private health insurance with one of the few insurance companies. About 10% of the population has private insurance, but often with rather limited coverage for benefits. Most private health insurance is a work-related benefit, and the premiums, which are usually age, sex and risk-related, are paid by employers.

Private health care can also be financed by the individual patient and approximately 20% of the private sector is financed in this way. In addition, more than half all terminations of pregnancy are carried out in the private sector. Other specialties where there is significant private practice include plastic surgery, psychotherapy and alternative medicine.

Hospitals are funded by the groups that purchase their services—mainly health authorities but also some direct fund-holding GPs. An allowance is paid by regions directly to teaching hospitals in recognition of their teaching and research costs. Certain specialised treatment centres and the Health Education Authority remain at present directly funded by the Department of Health.

Hospital specialists (consultants) are paid a salary determined by seniority and nationally agreed guidelines. They may be full or part time in the NHS: very few specialists work entirely in private practice. Private patients can be seen and treated in NHS hospitals. Hospitals make a charge for these facilities, but the calculation of cost is usually to the detriment of the health service.

Providers of care

Hospitals

Most hospitals, whether acute or long-stay, are managed by the health service and are thus not-for-profit. Of private sector hospitals, 60% are for-profit and the rest run by charitable organisations. There is no significant involvement of church organisations. About 60% of nursing homes for the elderly and people with mental or physical disability are also in the private sector.

Since the new NHS reforms, district health authorities 'purchase' health care from a range of facilities for their resident population. Hospitals and community services, as 'providers', are being established independently of district health authority control. Plans have to be approved by the Minister of Health. These 'trust' units have their own board of governors, can organise pay and service conditions for their staff and decide upon the services they provide.

Ambulatory care

GPs are self-employed and contract their services to the NHS: very few work privately. GPs are paid through a combination of capitation, items of service and a basic allowance. Capitation fees are enhanced for doctors practising in deprived areas, and there is also a higher fee for patients aged 75 or over. Item-of-service payments are paid for activities such as cervical screening, vaccinations and health promotion clinics. Quantitative targets of the proportion of the practice list screened must be reached in order for the doctor to be paid for some of these services.

A new initiative for fund-holding GPs allows some larger practices to buy certain hospital services directly, for example some surgical procedures. It is hoped that direct control of this portion of a patient's costs will give GPs incentives to choose higher quality of care.

A majority of doctors work in group practices and health centres with attached ancillary staff such as nurses, health visitors and midwives. These staff may be employed either by the practice or by the district health authority. GPs are reimbursed for the costs of staff they employ.

Patients have free choice of any GP within their area and are free to change GP if they wish. Equally, however, GPs can refuse to accept a patient or can discharge them. GPs usually have direct access to hospital facilities such as simple radiology and pathology, but referral to a consultant in the hospital outpatient department is needed for more specialised investigation. A patient can bypass the GP for admission to hospital if he attends a hospital accident and emergency department directly.

Public health

Public health developed in the UK during the middle of the nineteenth century. Until 1974, public health was practised in local authorities by the department of the medical officer of health. From 1974, this medical specialty, renamed community medicine, was transferred into the NHS. This reorganisation meant that certain local authority powers were lost. In 1990, the new name of public health medicine was adopted, but practised still from within the NHS.

Public health medicine

Public health doctors may be attached to a department of public health in a district or region, work in the national Department of Health or in an academic setting. The work varies from health needs assessment and evaluation of services to health education, medical manpower planning and service management. Some specialise in communicable disease control: these consultants work in close liaison with the non-medical environmental health officers attached to local authorities.

Undergraduate teaching

All medical schools have well-established public health departments and teach undergraduate students compulsory courses in public health. Subjects such as sociology and statistics are usually included during the first two (pre-clinical) years. In the fourth year subjects such as epidemiology and health promotion are brought in. These are all examined in university examinations. Students are, however, given little opportunity to experience the practice of public health medicine outside the classroom.

Postgraduate training

Training programmes are organised by regional health authorities and regulated by the Faculty of Public Health Medicine. Generally, doctors are expected to have completed at least two years post-registration in a clinical specialty before starting specialist training. Posts are awarded through competitive interview. The training programme is for five years. The first two include an academic course, either full or part time, leading to a written examination, Part I Membership of the Faculty of Public Health Medicine. This examination covers topics such as epidemiology, statistics, health services research, sociology, economics and management. During the following three years of higher specialist training, posts may be held in academic or service departments. During this period the second part of the membership examination must be passed. This consists of a written submission of about 20,000 words, based on work completed during training, and a viva examination.

Some opportunities for non-medical training in public health exist, for example in MSc courses at various institutes of public health or tropical medicine. However, there has been until recently a tendency to limit epidemiology courses and academic lecturer posts to medically qualified candidates. There is relatively little involvement of academic departments in the practical concerns of service public health departments.

4 | Financing health care

All 12 health systems of the EC seek to provide comprehensive health care financed through compulsory insurance of the majority of the population. Yet within EC countries this model differs significantly in that six of the countries, covering a majority of the total EC population, have legislation for a national health system.

A national health service implies a commitment to collective provision of health services; doctors in salaried and direct contractual employment; the majority of hospitals managed by public authorities; and finance through redistributive systems with a mixture of insurance and taxation. In contrast, the other six countries are more orientated towards individualised health care, with doctors more often in private practice (the 'liberal profession' model), hospitals more independent of public control, and health care financing with less public redistribution and control.

The six national health services in the EC have all developed since the second world war: the British NHS in 1948, the others during the 1960s and 1970s. The British, Danish and Italian national health services have GPs, who are independent contractors providing ambulatory and home care and mainly paid by list capitation, and hospital-based consultants who are salaried. The Greek and Portuguese national health services, however, are built around salaried GPs working from health centres and serving defined populations, while hospital care in Greece is still contracted as fee-for-service. The situation in Spain is complicated by the different stages of development of the regions, and is intermediate between these two models.

Comprehensive cover and care?

There continue to be different views of the level of benefits that compulsory health insurance or public funding should cover. In France, health insurance is compulsory for 99% of the resident population but does not cover the cost of all services. While inpatient care is free, ambulatory care costs are shared by copayments (an incentive against earlier discharge leading to the concept of 'hospital-at-home'). The non-profit 'mutuelles' have become entrepreneurial in filling this cost gap through a variety of secondary insurance schemes, which are of benefit to the patient but also evidence that copayments are more to do with reducing state expenditure than limiting 'excess' use.

In Germany, people in the top ten per cent of incomes are excluded by law from compulsory insurance. This is surprisingly like the nineteenth century medical view that, while insurance is acceptable for the poor, the rich should be charged directly as in traditional private practice.

Greece has a less visible system of private supplementation of public insurance. It is widely recognised that professionals, including doctors, escape paying taxes by not recording all their financial transactions. (Tax inspection is poorly organised and there is less tradition of paying taxes than in northern European countries.) It has been estimated that an extra 1% of the currently recognised gross national income could be being spent on health care in this way: but, of course, gross national product (GNP) itself would be larger if this 'black' economy was included.

Even countries with avowed national health systems are not uniform in ensuring full benefits to all people. For a start, all national health systems have some form of copayment, albeit usually modest. Copayments are charged on drugs prescribed in ambulatory care (but usually not in hospitals) in several countries. These arrangements vary, sometimes with an incentive of more copayment if the drug is regarded as 'less' beneficial. All countries make exemption for special groups, such as the elderly, people on low incomes, pregnant women and people with certain chronic illnesses. These exemptions are significant, in that it is such people who tend to be high users of pharmaceuticals. Thus the 'residual' group of people actually paying copayments may be less than half of all transactions, and call into question the purpose of the copayment.

Copayments are also frequently charged on services with a 'cosmetic' element—that is, spectacles, dental care and hearing aids. Again, certain groups gain exemption from the copayments, but the broader use of these services in the population and the relatively high proportion of copayment give them a significant place in the services. It is of note that one of the few positive findings of the RAND health insurance experiment in the USA was that copayments substantially reduced demand for dental care (Manning, Bailit, Benjamin and Newhouse 1986). Given the extent of dental disease in the population of Europe, EC countries (apart from Germany) appear to give a low priority to dental care for their populations.

A final area of copayments is for ambulatory or inpatient care. In France this is normal practice, but has been substantially offset by 'mutuelle' secondary insurance. In Italy the national health service is able to pay for care in private clinics and hospitals for some services if they are not readily available directly. Patients in private hospitals are able to receive 'hotel' benefits in these settings by extra payments, costs that better off people are now meeting through secondary insurance. In the UK, too, 'pay' beds in NHS hospitals allow better amenities within the public system. On the other hand, private health insurance in the UK usually pays for consultations and hospital care independently of NHS care.

How much spending on health care?

The traditional method of comparing the amount of health care spending in countries is to compare the proportion of GNP (the economist's term that indicates the total economic activity of a country, including earnings overseas). Thus it is a measure rather like income for an individual in society. It includes economic activity in both the private and public sectors.

Country spending on health care may be compared using per cent GNP which, in contrast to *per capita* expenditure, is not distorted by exchange rates. However, per cent GNP does not indicate the actual spending power; it is subject to inaccuracy in the denominator if there is a substantial 'black market' within the economy; and, because the total expenditure forms the numerator, it is important that similar elements of health care are included in the costs of all countries. This latter is important in costing uniformly social care, for example for elderly people ('nursing homes'), private medical care and complementary medicine.

In comparisons between large numbers of countries, there appears to be a correlation between increasing GNP and the increasing proportion spent on health care. This relationship is both cross-sectional, and also over time. The time series are relatively short, however, lasting the 30 years or so since the 1950s. In the 1960s, the developments of technological medicine led to new hospital building in all countries, rising numbers of staff per bed, and greater costs of investigations. It is also recognised that there is a relationship between supply and demand: where there are more doctors and more hospital beds, there tend to be higher admission rates.

In the 1980s, states have increasingly sought to intervene in the 'medical market' to limit the growth of medical care. The ways of doing this have mainly been to attempt to control supply—by manpower control (eg a *numerus clausus* for medical students, limitation of specialist appointments); by planning regulations for hospital building; and by increased influence over the financing systems. In contrast, the demand for medical care is less controllable: partly because the 'need' for health care is a professional assessment rather than a judgement by the patient (who depends on the professional both for identifying what is wrong and indicating what options there are for improvement); and partly because of the political difficulties of not responding to what patients 'want'.

Cost control by government has increased in all European health systems (Abel Smith 1992). Nevertheless, the organisation of financing within health services has an effect on total expenditure. At the system level, health services with centrally collected health funds, especially where they are voted through national representative bodies, tend to have greater control of total costs than fragmented insurance systems. At the hospital level, there is a hierarchy of control through payments, with annual budgets providing the greatest control, daily costs intermediate control and cost per case the least control. At the individual level, salaried payment of doctors is more likely to control costs than fee-for-service reimbursement.

The reason for these variations is that different financing schemes have different incentives for medical practice. Fee-for-service hospital practice (found, for example, in Belgium) encourages high throughput of patients (and thus high charges against insurance) but gives little incentive to non-interventional practice or prevention. Nevertheless, the public hospitals in most EC countries pay their doctors by salaries, thus choosing depth and range of clinical practice over throughput.

5 | Providers

The public/private divide

The history of hospital development in Europe is predominantly non-commercial. There has been a parallel development of private non-profit hospitals, run by self-help associations, ecclesiastic bodies and philanthropic foundations, with public hospitals usually built and run by local authorities for social and public health provision. In the latter category come fever hospitals, mental institutions and nursing homes for old people. Countries have varied in the distribution of provision for short-term patients, from the Netherlands and Germany where these are mainly provided by independent agencies to Italy where they are mainly state-owned and under the control of regional authorities.

The extent of private for-profit hospital care varies between countries. Private hospitals are banned by law in Belgium and the Netherlands. Denmark has only one private hospital, in Copenhagen. In the UK, private hospitals provide 5–10% of all beds, but patients attending private hospitals are mainly paying for themselves or through private insurance. In contrast, private non-profit and for-profit hospitals in Italy contract with the NHS for patients paid from public funds, although often charging a copayment to bring the hospital's income up from the level of NHS reimbursement to their full costs.

Private ambulatory care is much more widespread. In France and Germany, fee-for-service ambulatory care is paid through health insurance, and through private insurance in Britain. The emphasis on fee-for-service payment in Germany, France and Belgium has led to more specialisation than elsewhere. Denmark, Britain and Italy have retained general practice (paid by capitation), which reduces the need for specialist consultation. Spain, Portugal and Greece are also seeking to develop general practice, and thus limit specialisation with its attendant higher costs, although these countries have ex-perimented with salaried primary care doctors.

The extent of specialisation is substantially determined by the country's arrangements for professional referral. In countries where general practice is well established (Britain, Denmark, Italy, Netherlands) patients usually attend their GP, who then decides whether to refer the patient for a specialist's opinion or care. (In whether to refer the patient for a specialist's opinion or care. (In Italy, specialists are not allowed to refer patients between each other: they must always refer the patient back to the GP.) These countries do have some small areas of practice where patients can refer themselves to specialists, for example in accident care, sexually transmitted diseases and family planning. In France and Spain patients may go to a GP first, or refer themselves directly to a specialist.

The division between ambulatory and hospital care is absolute in Germany because of the financing system. Doctors must work in one or other sector, and are not allowed to work in both. This has led to the development of more day-case procedures than in other countries, but also to a tendency to repeat investigations in the two settings. In France and Belgium, specialists see patients in their private clinics and may admit them to hospital. In both Britain and Italy, GPs refer patients for assessment by a specialist: in Britain this is usually in a hospital outpatient department, in Italy it is usually at a local 'polyclinic' for ambulatory care. However, Italy is introducing incentives to hospital doctors to provide more outpatient care, because it is believed that the combined hospital and ambulatory care setting provides the best level of expertise.

Another aspect of variation between countries is the difference between health and social care. The boundary is of particular concern in caring for people with long-term disabilities, for example mental illness, physical handicap or disability in old age. Countries differ in their means of financing and organising care, both for institutional provision and community care. In practical terms, there are difficulties in all countries in the political and management interface between health, social and voluntary services, and it is important to be aware of the different agencies providing similar services when comparing statistics between countries.

Access to health care in European Community countries

EC citizens are covered by a reciprocal agreement between member countries to provide access to urgent medical treatment on the same basis as nationals of the member state being visited. Travellers can obtain a certificate of entitlement to emergency treatment in all EC countries before leaving their own country. In Britain, this form is available from post offices, but must be completed, stamped and signed by the counter official before leaving the country.

In some EC countries, charges are made at the time of treatment. An application for reimbursement must be made to the local sickness insurance fund before leaving the country. Failure to follow the correct procedure will forfeit the fees charged. Claims left until returning home are subject to delay, and may not be accepted. Because of the complexities, and because there are variations in the extent of cover between different EC countries, the European Commission still recommends that travellers should consider taking out medical insurance when going abroad.

These arrangements are unsatisfactory, and are open to abuse by local agencies directing travellers towards private health care rather than the public system. The EC could move towards introducing personal cards similar to an international driving licence, whereby a visitor can be readily identified and reimbursements become the responsibility of the host country's public sickness insurance rather than requiring the individual to negotiate with a bureaucracy in another country.

6 | Health commissioning

The health systems of EC countries are similar in having well developed mechanisms for funding and substantial provision. The countries differ, however, in their ability to use these structures to initiate broad policies which will maximise the population's health—an approach which may be termed health commissioning.

All EC health systems operate within a framework of national law. In some countries, such as Britain and Denmark, the state is clearly visible as a regulator and provider of services. In others, such as Belgium and Luxembourg, legislation creates an environment in which doctors, hospitals and insurance agencies operate with less visible state intervention.

While health care contributes to some aspects of health, especially in the acute treatment of suffering and the limitation of chronic illness, health is also determined by genetic, environmental and social factors. This is increasingly being acknowledged through the development of the World Health Organisation (WHO) *Health for All* initiative, and the European Healthy Cities programme.

The ability of health services to co-operate with other agencies varies, but it is less where there is little formal control, beyond legislation, of the health system itself. All European states have endorsed the *Health for All* charter, but there is great variation in implementation in national and local policies. Healthy Cities projects exist in all EC countries, but they vary in how much they are integrated with ordinary medical care services. It is easier for a public health department in a local authority to extend its range of concerns to other local government issues—environment, leisure, social care, housing—than it is to engage a fragmented health system of financing and providing agencies in similar developments.

The state is involved in the health system in three ways: as legal regulator of the arrangements for patients to receive medical care and doctors to receive remuneration; as contributor to health care financing either through formal taxes or through quasi-taxes such as compulsory social insurance; and as a guardian to ensure that the correct balance of resources is used to achieve optimum population health.

Health care may be conceived in an economic framework as an exchange of goods. Patients seeking medical care are making demands, while doctors providing services are supplying services. However, there are ways other than medical treatment of using resources to improve population health, and the priorities of medical practice, emphasising technical over social models of care, do not always provide optimal health benefits. There is thus a role in all health systems for an overview of resource allocation, health policy and population health outcomes—the task of 'health commissioning'.

The WHO *Health for All* programme has identified 38 targets for improving health and health care. Within the European region of WHO these have been accepted by individual govern-ments and incorporated in a strategy. Policies on how the population's health can be maximised, using the nation's resources as well as possible, are the responsibility of a government's Ministry of Health. Achieving these targets requires a range of actions by governments, by public participation, by local health services, by individual professionals. For policies to be carried out, there has to be some form of regional or district overview to decide on local health policies and resource use.

The concept of health commissioning has developed in Britain as a result of recent NHS changes. The new NHS structure requires publicly accountable bodies (health authorities) to use health financing resources available for the population to maximise health. Part of these resources can be used to develop co-operation between the health care and other sectors, including local authority and voluntary bodies. Most of the resources are used to pay contracts to health care providers of both primary and secondary care. The structure allows both a broad view of health care within the broader framework of *The Health of the Nation* (Department of Health 1992) and the European WHO Healthy Cities programme, and also a view on the balance of health services to be purchased across the range of health care.

Consumer knowledge and participation

The characteristic that prevents medical care becoming an ordinary market, from an economic viewpoint, is that the receivers of services are often unable to make informed choices about care.

Patients make many of the key choices of the health care system—whether their feelings and symptoms indicate that they are ill, and whether to consult a doctor. Population studies show there are wide variations in these choices between different people; one person will stoically accept symptoms that would lead another to consult a doctor immediately. Once a patient consults, good communication between doctor and patient should lead to a joint decision. But the key information—diagnosis, prognosis, treatment, implications—is in the hands of the doctor.

Yet doctors themselves do not perform uniformly. Different doctors vary in their action when faced with similar patients, and an individual doctor makes different decisions for patients with similar conditions. Thus, doctors operate a threshold for care. This threshold, both individually and collectively, is affected by knowledge and supply. Medical knowledge can lead to choices either to act or not to act.

These aggregate decisions on thresholds to medical care determine spending on health care. In both national health services and social insurance systems doctors are gatekeepers to resources: they legitimise a patient's claim for services. Country health systems seek to influence doctors' decisions broadly, for example in availablity of services (hospitals, drugs), and specifically, for example in the level of remuneration given to particular services. (When notification of infectious diseases was regarded to be of considerable importance, the fees provided to doctors for notification were relatively higher than they are at present.)

Public health medicine—current practice

Public health is the science and art of preventing disease, prolonging life and promoting health through organised efforts of society. Public health medicine is that branch of medicine which specialises in public health. Its chief responsibilities are the surveillance of the health of a population, the identification of its health needs, the fostering of policies which promote health, and the evaluation of health services (Acheson 1988).

Public health medicine practice in EC countries varies, as a result both of the organisation of political structures and of the financing and managerial control of the health systems. The range of public health medicine practice includes:

- *Communicable disease control and environmental health.*
  In all EC countries, doctors trained in public health medicine are available to give advice to central and local governments on the control of communicable diseases. The AIDS epidemic of the 1980s has increased concern about this responsibility. In

countries such as Denmark, Germany and Greece, the public health doctor responsible for environmental control is employed by the local authority (eg municipal or provincial council). In other countries, for example, the UK, Italy and Portugal, the doctor is administratively within the health service while in practice working closely with local authority colleagues.

- *Services for special care groups (eg children, mentally and physically handicapped, elderly, etc)*
  In many European countries, such as Ireland, Portugal and Denmark, services for these special care groups are managed by public health physicians. Co-ordination with social services is also needed. In Germany, almost all personal health services have been passed to contracting doctors in specialist practice. In Britain and the Netherlands these services are increasingly being managed by specialists working across the hospital/community interface.

- *Health service resource use*
  In France and Spain, doctors may be employed by sickness insurance agencies to give broad advice on the distribution of funds. In the UK, public health physicians contribute to decisions on the allocation of resources within the NHS. In some countries such as Netherlands and Germany, there is practice of individual 'insurance medicine', in which doctors see patients to consider the appropriateness of clinical decisions and insurance payments.

- *Planning and management*
  Several health systems have regional and district levels for administration below the central Ministry of Health. In some countries, such as Italy and the UK, doctors with a training in public health medicine may take administrative positions within these decentralised authorities, and also as directors of hospitals. In other countries there is a clear professional separation between doctors and administrators.

- *Research and development, education and training*
  All EC countries except Luxembourg have at least one academic institute of public health undertaking research and education. Also, universities, working in multidisciplinary settings, are increasingly concerned with research and policy issues in public health.

The task of the public health physician is to make a medical contribution to the following activities:

- To use epidemiological methods to:
  —define and describe the health needs of the population
  —identify environmental and social hazards to health
  —elucidate the causes and determinants of disease

- To provide advice to those concerned with setting of priorities and planning services

- To participate in developing policy on disease prevention, health promotion and health education

- To undertake surveillance of communicable and non-communicable disease and co-ordinate disease control activities

- To evaluate the implementation and outcome (effectiveness and efficiency) of health policies and services provided in populations.

In all EC countries, public health medicine must be introduced into a variety of settings to be effective: through the local public health department; through the insurance funds; and through hospital and other health service administration. The challenge for all countries is to be able to monitor and influence the health service of a local population and to be able to demonstrate perceptible health gains. To achieve this, countries will need to be able systematically to review health information for the population; ensure co-ordination between the different sectors of the health system; and assess and improve the efficiency and effectiveness of health care.

These tasks require different inputs in different health systems. A way forward can be the preparation of a report on the health of the population which will spell out the areas of unmet need, inefficient provision and opportunities for more effective resource use. This work may be done in association with university departments of public health, which may have specific expertise in information analysis, but the report must be capable of affecting the health system directly. Preparing the report and ensuring change as a result is the work of public health medicine.

Public health medicine in the European Community

From 1975 the EC has required mutual recognition of specialties within member countries, but the actual arrangements for specialty training and accreditation are determined individually in each EC country. In France, for instance, specialty training starts before the end of the undergraduate period, and doctors must comply with specialty regulations of attachment to specialist departments as well as general clinical experience. In Italy and Germany doctors apply for part-time specialist training programmes within university departments some years after graduation. In the UK, the GMC delegates accreditation of specialist training to the Joint Committee on Higher Medical Training, a body which also controls the final number of consultants by approving only a limited number of junior staff positions.

Specialty accreditation for public health medicine must take place within these arrangements that are specific for each country. There is often an important role for a national school of public health (for example Portugal, Greece) but, increasingly, other university departments are also involved in teaching. Academic training for public health medicine appears to be better developed than the arrangements for in-service practical training. In some countries, for example the Netherlands and Italy, public health departments usually employ their medical staff and second them for academic training. In other countries, for example France and Spain, it is possible to work within the field of public health medicine with less academic training.

There is, in all countries, some separation in practice between university and health service practitioners of public health medicine. This is partly because epidemiological studies do not need direct patient contact, and can therefore be undertaken independently of the health service. It is also because health service managers and administrative bodies do not always understand how to use epidemiological and evaluative skills effectively. Closer working between university departments and public health physicians in administrative and fieldwork positions will be a crucial step for the firm establishment of the specialty.

There are also difficulties in the use of words in translation. Thus, in the Netherlands there is a broad specialisation of 'social medicine' which encompasses four sub-specialties of general health care (closest to public health medicine), insurance medicine, occupational medicine and child health. In contrast, in Denmark 'social medicine' is one of three branches within public health medicine, which also embraces environmental and administrative medicine.

Developing a European specialty of public health medicine

Under the 1975 directive of the Commission of the European Community, and subsequent modifications, each member state must give the same legal recognition to 'formal qualifications in specialist medicine' awarded in other member countries as they give their own. But neither the UK nor Ireland give any legal recognition to specialist status, and other member states do not recognise public health medicine as a specialty under the directive. Thus, at present, the directive has no practical effect in relation to public health medicine.

One way forward for mutual recognition would be for the remaining member states to seek recognition of the specialty under the directive. Any qualification to be included would have to be awarded by the 'competent authority' recognised by the directive (eg for Germany by the Landesärztekammern, for Belgium by the Minister for Public Health). It would also have to meet the standards, set in a second directive, of a minimum of four years 'practical and theoretical instruction', undertaken 'in a university centre, in a teaching hospital or, where appropriate, in a health establishment approved for the purpose by the competent authorities' and involving 'the personal participation of the doctor training to be a specialist in the activity and in the responsibilities of the establishments concerned'.

Another way forward would be for two or more member countries to put forward to the European Commission proposals for a directive on specific training for public health medicine. If introduced, such a directive would go beyond the broadly defined requirements of the current directive on medical training and seek to establish more precise and detailed standards specific to training in public health medicine. It would also make these mandatory for anyone wishing to take up practice in the specialty, thus overcoming the weakness in the UK and Ireland of the current directive on mutual recognition of medical qualifications.

Conclusion

The increasing economic and political links between the member countries of the EC are also likely to have implications for health systems. While the Community Treaties do not cover the health field broadly, 'public health' is being recognised as within the competence of the Commission, and there is in-creasing concern to ensure uniform arrangements for medical specialties within the framework of free movement of workers.

Public health medicine is needed within the health systems of all European countries to ensure a population approach to the provision and outcome of health services, and an appropriate balance between direct health care and other ways—environmental, social or educational—to achieve health. Public health medicine can make an important contribution to this process. It is thus important for public health medicine to be recognised within the movement for medical specialty recognition in the EC. A common structure for the development of public health medicine training and practice in EC countries could help develop a population approach in all EC health systems, and see significant improvements in the population's health through health services, prevention, public health policies, and research and development.

7 | Towards European integrations

Comparisons

The prospect of a single market and increasing political harmonisation within the EC, will inevitably have repercussions for the health systems of EC states. A conference held in Rotterdam in 1988 on the theme of competition in health care reports the views of a range of commentators from EC countries (Casparie, Hermans and Paelink 1990). As the political process develops, the opportunities for change and harmonisation will become more clear. The present report is only a 'snapshot' of a dynamic process that needs continuing attention.

The OECD has collected data and provided commentaries on the differences and trends in health systems of a range of industrialised countries (OECD 1990). Inferences from these data need to be tempered by an understanding of their limitations, as data collected in different countries frequently do not measure the same things. For example, 'hospital beds' in one country may include nursing home beds for elderly people and exclude them in another, perhaps because of differences in financing. The number of doctors in a country may be recorded by the professional organisation or by the main employing agents—giving substantially different results. The costs of hospital doctors are usually included (as salaries) in European countries but excluded (as private fees) in the USA. Further limitations are that the existing data give little information on how the different structural parts of the health system interact, or on the outcomes of health care.

Economically, spending on health care appears to behave in the same way as 'luxury' goods: the proportion of GNP spent on health care tends to rise with GNP. But these broad figures hide surprising differences between countries. Culyer (in OECD 1990) noted that in 1983 the USA was 40% richer and the Federal Republic of Germany 15% richer than the UK. Yet, compared per capita with the UK, the USA had 60% more doctors and Germany 85% more; the USA had 27% fewer beds while Germany had 40% more; and both countries had fewer nurses—30% fewer in the USA and 59% fewer in Germany. These differences may be partly due to different recording systems, but also reflect different styles of health practice and different financial incentives. Health care cost differences reflect different staff levels, staff incomes utilisation by patients but bear little relationship to health care needs between countries except for the important broad determinant of age structure.

The USA is frequently used as a comparison country, particularly because of its leading economic position. Yet the USA health system is markedly different from those in the EC countries. For example, most European countries showed a rising pattern of expenditure on health care (indicated by the percentage of GNP spent) during the 1970s and a flattening in the 1980s. In contrast, the proportion of GNP spending on health care in the USA in the 1980s continued to rise. The small proportion, around 40%, of health care expenditure that comes from public funds in the USA is in marked contrast to the European average of around 80%.

Enthoven (in OECD 1990) has summarised the major deficiencies of the health system of the USA. In financing health care, a system dominated by private medical practice, 35 million Americans - about one in six people - have no health care insurance or protection against medical expenses. 'Millions more have inadequate coverage that leaves them exposed to large risks or to exclusions for care of pre-existing conditions.' Tax relief on employer-paid health insurance, predominantly going to higher-income families, costs the federal government more than the federal budget available for Medicaid (medical expenses support for low-income people).

In provision of health care in the USA, there are high rates of technological interventions, for example coronary artery bypass grafts, but these often take place in small hospitals with low activity rates and consequently high mortalities. Surveys of clinical practice, based on consensus standards, show that these interventions are frequently 'inappropriate' or 'equivocal'. Yet the infant mortality rate is higher than in most western European countries. Most worrying of all, the public do not support the system they have got, but politicians are unable to legislate a fairer or more efficient system because it would offend the existing powerful vested interests.

After reviewing the limitations of health care in the USA, Evans and Barer (in OECD 1990) identify three critical aspects that must be protected in European health systems:

- the global controls on health spending, in both public and private sectors, in line with national economic policies;
- the clear separation of individual contributions for health care from the experience of illness or health status;

- the existing universal financing and co-ordinated delivery of health care.

Reinhardt (in OECD 1990) summarised contrasting models of control of health systems in the USA and Europe, respectively, in viewing the USA as 'micromanagement' and European countries as 'macromanagement'. In the USA, individual consumers (or alliances, such as Health Maintenance Organisations) are pitted against providers of health care, who are also relatively small, competing units (private practice physicians and hospitals). In European countries, the demands of patients are controlled through pre-determined budgets, while providers are regulated through national and regional planning. Without giving up the advantages of the European systems described by Evans and Barer (above), a middle ground, taking advantages from both models, may be to develop 'managed markets'—as, for example in the reformed UK NHS.

Perhaps the most important factor controlling the development of European health systems in the 1990s will be the power of consumers. Governments can create regulations for financing and providing health care which ensure that all citizens have access and that services achieve agreed minimum standards. But further improvements will depend on the concern, and power, of consumers to demand changes locally. This will include alliances of consumers into patient groups, understanding of the health system's management arrangements, and seeking public forums to increase political pressure for change. The response of the British and French governments to the demands of people with haemophilia who contracted AIDS may be an example.

Title X in the Treaty of Maastricht, 1992

The EC made a major step towards further integration at the December 1991 Maastricht summit and the subsequent February 1992 Treaty signing of new articles. While health issues have not, heretofore, been a clear responsibility for the Community, the new Title X is specifically entitled Public Health. It is worth reproducing the Title in full:

'Title X

Public Health

Article 129

1. The Community shall contribute towards ensuring a high level of human health protection by encouraging co-operation between the Member States and, if necessary, lending support to their action.

Community action shall be directed towards prevention of disease, in particular the major health scourges, including drug dependence, by promoting research into their causes and transmission, as well as health information and education.

Health protection requirements shall form a constituent part of the Community's other policies.

2. Member states shall, in liaison with the Commission, co-ordinate among themselves their policies and programmes in the areas referred to in paragraph 1. The Commission may, in close contact with the Member States, take any useful initiative to promote such co-ordination.

3. The Community and the Member States shall foster co-operation with third countries and competent international organisations in the sphere of public health.

4. In accordance to contribute to the achievement of the objectives referred to in this Article, the Council:

—in accordance with the procedure in Article 189b and after consulting the Economic and Social Committee and the Committee of the Regions, shall adopt incentive measures, excluding any harmonisation of the laws and regulations of the Member States;

—acting by qualified majority on a proposal by the Commission, shall adopt recommendations.'

Paragraph 4 clearly excludes 'harmonisation of the laws and regulations of the Member States' as a means of achieving public health. However, the specific exclusion allows all other ways to be possible. 'Incentive measures' in EC code usually means finance, including programme grants, training fellowships, research support, as well as meetings and publications. Until now, these have been available only for identified fields, particularly AIDS and cancer. The regulations henceforth are much more general, and the opportunity for proposing EC action in public health is greatly strengthened.

But what is public health in the view of the EC? First, it is 'health protection', and there shall be co-operation between member states to achieve it. A wide range of environmental health issues, from air pollution to accidents, may be included. This could give a major lift to collaboration on *Health for All* and Healthy Cities work.

Second, prevention of disease, health information and health education are specified. These are, of course, all component parts of the health services of member states, so that the public health chapter of the Treaty has brought EC competence directly into health systems. Prevention is part of medical practice daily, from cervical screening to check-ups for elderly people. And there will surely be much discussion about which health problems can count as a 'major scourge'.

Third, paragraph 1 ensures that health implications are taken into account in all other EC policies. This could have major economic implications, not just for immediate issues such as the subsidies given to tobacco farming in southern states but also for nutritional policies, transport and the environment more broadly.

Conclusion

There are variations between the health systems of EC states, although these differences are less than between European countries and the USA. Health care is a major factor—between 5 and 10%—of European economic activity. It has been mainly ignored up to now. While health systems are formally outside the competence of the EC, it is likely that, as the states draw closer together, there will be a trend towards greater similarity also between health systems. Factors towards harmonisation include the development of single insurance markets, pressure from employers to align the costs and benefits of health protection, co-ordination of initiatives in disease prevention and, as information becomes more available, pressure from patients to have access to the same range and quality of services as citizens in other countries.

At present, European health systems can be divided broadly into 'national health services' and 'liberal profession' models. However, government regulation of costs and quality is increasing in all countries. A 'managed market' for health care may, in time, be seen as the best middle ground, allowing governments power of regulation without direct management responsibilities.

If the EC moves towards a managed market for health care, then the 1990 NHS reforms should provide a strong competitive position for the UK. As UK experience has shown, health system managers currently have less understanding of how to purchase health care effectively than of how to provide it. To ensure epidemiologically-based health needs assessment, purchasing policies that give due emphasis to health promotion and disease prevention as well as treatment and care, and to develop relevant and valid measures of the outcome, the EC needs to strengthen public health medicine within all its countries. In this, as in the larger sphere of the NHS, the UK has an important opportunity to lead.

References

Abel-Smith B. The history of medical care. In: Martin EW, ed: *Comparative development in social welfare*. London: Allen & Unwin, 1972

Abel-Smith B. *Cost containment and new priorities in the European Community*. Aldershot: Avebury, 1992

Abel-Smith B, Maynard A. *The organisation, financing and cost of health care in the European Community*. Brussels: Commission of the European Communities, 1979

Acheson ED (Chairman). *Public health in England. Report of the committee of inquiry into the future development of the public heath function*. London: HMSO, 1988

Alber J, Esping-Andersen G, Rainwater L. Studying the welfare state: issues and queries. In: Dierkes M, Weiler HN, Antal AB, eds: *Comparative policy research*. London: Gower-WZB Publications, 1987

British Medical Association. *European Communities, and European Community medical bodies. Information notes—Europe, 1 and 2*. London: BMA, 1991

Casparie AF, Hermans HEGM, Paelink JHP, eds. *Competitive health care in Europe*. Aldershot: Dartmouth, 1990

Department of Health. *The health of the nation*. London: HMSO, 1992

Duplessis P, Dab W, McCarthy M, Portella E, eds. *Public health and industrialised countries*. Quebec: Les Publications du Quebec, 1989

Field M, ed. *Success and crisis in national health systems: a comparative approach*. London: Routledge, 1989

Ham C, Robinson R, Benzeval M. *Health checks*. London: King's Fund Institute, 1990

Manning WG, Bailit HL, Benjamin B, Newhouse JP. *The demand for dental care*. Santa Monica, CA: The Rand Corporation, 1986 (RAND/R-3225-HHS)

Maxwell RJ. *Health and wealth: an international study of health-care spending*. Lexington, MA: Lexington Books, 1981

Maynard A. *Health care in the European Community*. London: Croom Helm, 1975

McCarthy M. *Evolution and implementation of the Italian health service reform of 1978*. London: Chadwick Press, 1992

McLachlan G, Maynard A, eds. *The public/private mix for health*. London: Nuffield Provincial Hospitals Trust, 1982

Committee on Choices in Health Care. *Choices in Health Care*. Rijswijk: Ministry of Welfare, Health and Cultural Affairs, 1992

Organisation for Economic Co-operation and Development. *Health care systems in transition*. Paris: OECD, 1990

Schneider M, Dennerlain RK-H, Köse A, Scholtes L, eds. Health care in the European Community member states. *Health Policy (Netherlands)* 1992; **20(1/2)**: 1–251